REFER TO OCCUPATIONAL THERAPY

REFER TO OCCUPATIONAL THERAPY

A.J. Shopland
P.M. Hardial
A.M. Unwin
S.M. Vickers
V.R. Westmore
A.J. Williams

Second Edition

CHURCHILL LIVINGSTONE
Edinburgh London and New York 1979

CHURCHILL LIVINGSTONE
Medical Division of Longman Group Limited

Distributed in the United States of America by Longman Inc., 19 West 44th Street, New York, N.Y. 10036, and by associated companies, branches and representatives throughout the world.

First Edition 1975
  Reprinted 1976
Second Edition 1979

ISBN 0 443 01866 9

British Library Cataloguing in Publication Data

Refer to occupational therapy. – 2nd Ed.
  1. Occupational therapy
  I. Shopland, Angela J
  615'.8515   RM735   78-41002

Printed in Hong Kong by
Wah Cheong Printing Press Ltd

PREFACE TO THE SECOND EDITION

Occupational therapy is one of the professions complementary to medicine. Occupational therapists, along with nurses, speech therapists, remedial gymnasts, physiotherapists and other paramedical staff, form the rehabilitation team whose aim is to return any person in their care to the greatest possible level of independence. This team integrates and overlaps in a constantly changing pattern depending on the personnel involved. The occupational therapist's individual role is that of functional assessment and graded activity. Each activity has the dual purpose of being part of a treatment programme and being interesting in itself so that a task is done because it is enjoyable as well as beneficial. Occupational therapists work with both the physically and mentally ill, but psychiatry is not included in this small notebook.

'Refer to Occupational Therapy' is an attempt to produce a checklist for physical treatments. The checklist format was adopted deliberately as being of maximum use for quick reference, hence the dual nature of its title. However, the authors wish to give a warning to those who have kept this book constantly in their uniform pockets. Checklists give confidence, jog memories and enable bridges to be built over mental blanks, but they are also inhibitors of original thought. The best users of this book are those who have realised its limitations and use it essentially for quick reference.

Occupational therapists need to adapt their basic knowledge continually. This book is a first stepping stone in a wide field in which no two treatment plans are ever the same.

CONTRIBUTORS

S.J. Berry; A. Billingham; S. Billingham; S. Capel; J. Clarke;
V.J. Collins; H.P. Cookson; B. Dahl; B.J. Davies; J.C. Duhig; J.
Gardener; G. Gillespie; J.A. Girling; D.J. Harmer; G.M. Hewett;
R. Higman; E.J. Hobson; S.K. Martin; L.M. Hooyveld; A.B.
Howard; E.M. Humphreys; S. Hunter; J.M. Jones; P.A. Kerr;
S.J. Lake; J.M. Lea; C.M. Newby; J.M. Newman; W.E.J. Nobbs;
J.L. Porter; L.A. Potter; R. Poyser; N.R. Price; P.A. Raynes; C.A.
Thompson; J. Tovey; E. Treglown; S.M. Tucker; P.E. Whiting;
J.A. Williams; C.M. Wilson; B.C. Morgan; A.T. Nijenhuis—
Joint Measurement.

ACKNOWLEDGEMENTS

With thanks to the following hospitals, from which valuable
information was gathered during hospital practice:
Farnham Park Rehabilitation Centre
Frenchay Hospital
Hillingdon Hospital
The London Hospital
Medway Hospital
The National Hospital
New Cross Hospital
Poole General Hospital
Queen Alexandra Hospital
St. Helier Hospital
St. James' Hospital, Kent
Wolfson Medical Rehabilitation Centre
Whipps Cross Hospital
With special thanks to Miss K.M. Ingamells M.A.O.T., T.Dip.
(Vice principal of St. Loyes school of Occupational Therapy) for
her help and guidance in compiling this book.

CHAPTERS

1 / UPPER LIMB INJURIES

SHOULDER INJURIES

Types
Fractured neck of humerus
Fractured tuberosity of humerus
Fractured shaft of humerus
Fractured scapula
Capsulitis
Tendonitis
Ruptured supra-spinatus tendon
Dislocated shoulder.

Fractured neck of humerus or tuberosity

Immobilisation
Plaster of Paris (P.O.P.) over the shoulder joint with the elbow
   set at 90° for 4-6 weeks
Adduction fracture set in abduction
Abduction fracture set in adduction.

An impacted fracture is slung and movement is started
   immediately.

Fractured shaft of humerus

Immobilisation
P.O.P., 'U' slab or back slab over the shoulder with the elbow
   set at 90° for 5-7 weeks

Delayed union
Continue immobilisation for 10 weeks or internally fixate with
   a plate along the humerus or kuntchner nail down shaft.

9

Complication
Radial nerve involvement.

Fractured scapula

Immobilisation
Strapping/sling for 1-3 weeks.

Dislocated shoulder

Medical treatment
Anterior dislocation:
   Kocher's manipulation
   Arm immobilised in a sling.
Posterior dislocation:
   Hippocrates reduction
   Arm immobilised in a sling.
Recurrent dislocation:
(a) When the glenoid cavity is at fault the Bankart's
    operation is carried out to deepen the cavity or re-attach
    capsule to glenoid ring
(b) If the capsule is weak a Putti Platt operation is
    performed to shorten subscapularis and the anterior
    fibres of the capsule to limit lateral rotation. The limb is
    then bandaged to the trunk for 4 weeks.

Precautions
Recurrent dislocation. Shoulder must be strengthened. Do not
  give rotation exercises until the last stage of treatment.

Complications of a shoulder injury
Capsulitis (frozen shoulder)
Deltoid palsy
Brachial plexus lesion.

Aims of treatment
1 Stabilise
2 Mobilise
3 Independence in dressing and personal care

4 Functional assessment, e.g. hanging up coat; combing hair; tying apron; tucking in shirt.

Early stage
Principles of occupational therapy:
1 Always treat in a sprung sling or O.B. Help Arm
2 Give gentle flexion and abduction exercises
3 Give wide, bilateral movements to prevent compensation
4 Upgrade activities by weakening springs or reducing weights.

Activities
One week daily:
1 Bi-lateral sanding
2 Stool seating
3 Weaving unadapted at table height
4 Polishing a table top
5 Games: span game (upgrade by using increased lengths of dowelling); draughts; solitaire
6 Cooking, e.g. rolling pastry in a sprung sling
7 Work given to patient when prone on bed or table. The shoulder automatically falls into 90° of flexion. Games can be played, e.g. draughts

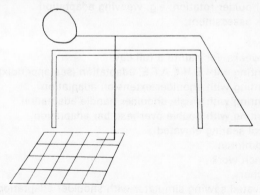

Figure 1

8 Dressing practice.

Middle stage
Principles of occupational therapy:
1 Work for flexion and abduction
2 Give bilateral activities to avoid compensation.

Activities
Two weeks daily:
   1 Bi-lateral sanding
   2 Printing unadapted
   3 Printing with the double overhead bar adaptation
   4 Printing with the single shoulder handle adaptation
   5 Stool seating
   6 Elevated sawing simulator with shoulder adaptation
   7 Light benchwork: planing and sawing
   8 Domestic work: cleaning windows; washing; ironing
   9 Games: quoits; table tennis; skittles
  10 Weaving on a rug loom
  11 Guillotining.

Late stage
Principles of occupational therapy;
1 Work for flexion, abduction and rotation
2 Fix the arm in a sling with the shoulder at 90° of abduction
   for shoulder rotation, e.g. weaving adaptation
3 Work assessment.

Activities
Three weeks, for half to a full day:
   1 Printing with S.H.E.A.F.E. adaptation (see appendix)
   2 Printing with shoulder extension adaptation
   3 Printing with single shoulder handle adaptation
   4 Printing with double overhead bar adaptation
   5 Stool seating elevated
   6 Badminton
   7 Bench work
   8 Archery
   9 Elevated sawing simulator with shoulder adaptation
  10 Gardening
  11 Cross cut sawing

12 Cement mixing

13 Housework: washing curtains and hanging out; bread making/cake beating

14 Weaving adapted with arms fixed to give rotation

15 Work simulation.

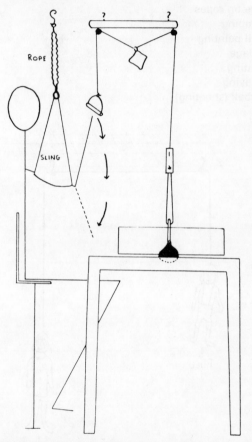

ROPE

SLING

Figure 2 Adaptation for internal and external rotation

N.B. A frozen shoulder can take up to three months to recover.

Suggested activities for children

1 Table tennis
2 Quoits
3 Skittles
4 Cooking
5 Toys on ropes
6 Climbing
7 Wall painting
8 Collage
9 Printing
10 Weaving
11 Netball (shooting).

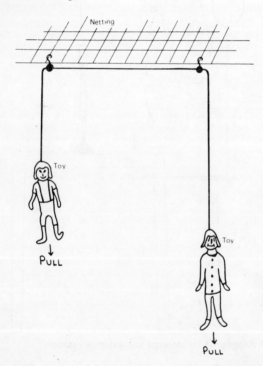

Figure 3

Other treatment for shoulder injuries

Physiotherapy - for relief of pain, stability and mobility

Remedial gym - to build up strength and increase range of movement.

ELBOW INJURIES AND CONDITIONS

Types

Supracondylar fracture

Fractured olecranon

Fractured head of radius

Tennis elbow

Golfer's elbow

Fracture dislocations

Rheumatoid arthritis.

Supracondylar fracture

Immobilisation

P.O.P. for three weeks or a collar and cuff or St John's sling with the elbow at an acute angle (especially with children).

Fractured olecranon

Immobilisation

P.O.P. with the elbow in 90° of flexion, for 2-3 weeks. The shoulder and wrist are often included in the P.O.P.

Internal fixation is often necessary.

With gross displacement of the fractured olecranon, it often travels up the humerus because of the strength of triceps. In such a case the olecranon will be excised and triceps replaced. The limb is then immobilised in P.O.P. for approximately 4 weeks with the elbow in 90-100° flexion.

Fractured head of radius

If the fracture is severe, the head of radius is excised.

If it is simple, the elbow is immobilised in a sling for 2 days to one week. Movement is started as soon as possible.

Tennis elbow

Tennis elbow is due to tendonitis of the common extensor origin. The elbow is strapped or slung, or immobilised in P.O.P. for up to 10 days.

Dislocation of elbow

Immobilisation

Gentle traction followed by P.O.P. for three weeks with the elbow in 90° of flexion.

Precautions and complications

1 Ulnar nerve involvement
2 Frozen shoulder (capsulitis)
3 Volkmann's ischaemic contracture
4 Avoid passive extension as this can lead to myositis ossificans.

Myositis ossificans

Due to tearing of the periosteum leading to displacement of osteoblasts into the muscle, resulting in ossification
Treatment:
Immobilisation for 6-8 weeks followed by gentle active treatment
Surgery if necessary to excise calcification followed by immobilisation for 6-8 weeks, then gentle active treatment.

Aims of treatment

1 Mobilise: first flexion and extension; pronation and supination, and grip
2 Functional assessment: check other joints; hand, wrist and shoulder
3 Personal independence
4 Strengthen.

Early stage

Principles of occupational therapy:
1 Work for flexion and extension—pushing rather than reaching

2 Work for mobility rather than stability
3 Stress to the patient not to passively extend the elbow, e.g. by carrying heavy shopping bag
4 A.D.L. check.

Activities
1-2 weeks, daily:
  1 Weaving with flexion and extension adaptations
  2 Weaving with F.E.P.S. adaptation for pronation and supination, and grip
  3 Washing and ironing small items
  4 Cooking: pastry and dough rolling
  5 Wire twister for pronation, supination and grip
  6 Games: wall solitaire; table tennis; draughts; bagatelle with a long pole
  7 Light gardening: hoeing; weeding; using a trowel
  8 Elevated sawing simulator
  9 Stool seating
10 Painting
11 Polishing
12 Window cleaning
13 Printing unadapted.

Middle stage

Activities
2 weeks daily:
  1 Printing with S.H.E.A.F.E. adaptation
  2 Printing with double overhead bar adaptation
  3 Printing with low double overhead bar to give elbow extension
  4 Weaving on a rug loom
  5 Electric drill with an overhead handle
  6 Wire twister with a long handle
  7 Light sawing
  8 Making coat hangers on a jig
  9 Archery
10 Washing: sheets, curtains, towels
11 Gardening: digging

12 Games: quoits; tennis; badminton
13 Benchwork: screwdriving included.

Last stage

Activities

1-2 weeks daily:

1 Cross cut sawing
2 Bench work
3 Lathe work if strength needed
4 Cement mixing if strength needed
5 Scaffolding if strength needed
6 Work simulation
7 Wrought iron work.

Suggested activities for children

1 Skittles
2 Bagatelle
3 Hoop-la
4 Darts: last stage
5 Table tennis
6 Gardening
7 Basic cooking: rolling pastry
8 Toys to be wound with keys
9 Football game (for pronation and supination)
10 Weaving.

Upgrade and adapt where necessary.

WRIST INJURIES AND CONDITIONS

Types

Fractures of the radius and ulna (including Smith's and Colles fractures)
Fractures of the carpal bones
Carpal tunnel syndrome (usually median nerve compression)
Crush injuries

Tendon injuries
Rheumatoid arthritis
Nerve injuries.

Fractured radius and ulna—mid-third

Immobilisation
P.O.P. from axilla to metacarpo-phalangeal (M.C.P.) heads with
the elbow in 90° of flexion, for 10-12 weeks.

The fracture is often slow to unite so it is often internally
fixed.

Fractured radius and ulna—lower third

Immobilisation
P.O.P. from above elbow to M.C.P. heads with the elbow in
90° of flexion, for 4 weeks.

Internal fixation is often necessary.

Monteggia complication
Fractured lower third of ulna with dislocation of the radius.
Usually internally fixed.

Fractured lower third of radius—Colles or Smith's fracture

Immobilisation
P.O.P. from below elbow to M.C.P heads, for 5 weeks.

Complications
Sudeck's atrophy
Rupture of extensor pollicis longus tendon
Oedema
There is often slow recovery due to poor blood supply to the
wrist
Cross union is a possible complication in all fractures of
radius and ulna if not internally fixed.

Aims of treatment
1. Increase and strengthen grip

2 Mobilise; first flexion and extension and then pronation and supination
3 Functionally assess other joints: hand, elbow and shoulder
4 Sensory assessment
5 Work assessment.

Activities

Early stage
Treatment daily:
 1 Printing with F.E.P.S. adaptation
 2 Weaving with F.E.P.S. adaptation
 3 Wire twisting machine for flexion and extension, pronation and supination
 4 Clay work
 5 Games: span game; water syphon; light quoits; peggotty
 6 Sanding curved surfaces
 7 Using a surform on curved surfaces
 8 Rolling out pastry
 9 Polishing
10 Cord knotting
11 Stereognosis testing.

Middle stage
Treatment daily:
 1 Printing/weaving with F.E.P.S. adaptation
 2 Spoke shaving
 3 Wire twister for grip, and pronation and supination
 4 Pronation and supination football
 5 Sawing to increase strength
 6 Printing with wooden disc adaptation for active wrist extension; see Fig. 63
 7 Bread making: mixing and beating
 8 Laundry: wringing out clothes
 9 Using a screwdriver
10 Darts
11 Quoits: heavy weight
12 Cutting with scissors
13 Painting with a large brush.

Last stage
Treatment daily:
1 Volley ball
2 Badminton
3 Heavy gardening
4 Use of shears
5 Brick laying
6 Heavy washing: towels, curtains, sheets
7 Netball (shooting)
8 Bench work: sawing, hammering, planing
9 Wrought iron work
10 Use of mortise and tenon machine
11 Lathe work for static grip.

Length of treatment
The length of treatment will vary according to the age of the
    patient and the severity of the fracture.

Carpal tunnel syndrome
This condition results from swelling of the synovial sheaths of
    the flexor tendons where they pass beneath the flexor
    retinaculum. The median nerve which accompanies them
    becomes compressed as the walls of the 'tunnel' are
    unyielding.

Signs and symptoms
Paraesthesia in the median nerve distribution
Pain at night
Weakness and stiffness in the hand
Wasting of the thenar eminence.

Precautions
Diminished sensation.

Aims of treatment
1 General strengthening and mobilisation
2 Sensation training.

Functional assessment
1 Grip measurement with dynomometer

2 Sensation testing.

Prognosis
Following decompression, good.

Length of treatment
One hour daily for 1 to 2 weeks.

Other treatment
Drug therapy, e.g. hydrocortisone injection
Surgery
Night splintage.

2 / LOWER LIMB INJURIES

HIP INJURIES AND CONDITIONS

Types
Fractured neck of femur
Fractured shaft of femur
Osteo-arthrosis of the hip
Dislocation of the hip.

Fractured neck of femur

Possible treatment
  (a) Internal fixation with pin and plate, e.g. Smith Peterson
  (b) Replacement of head of femur, e.g. Austen Moore or
      Thompson femoral components
  (c) Total hip replacement, e.g. Charnley low friction
      arthroplasty if osteo arthrosis affects hip joint as a result
      of a fracture or other trauma; or if Austen Moore or
      Thompson components worn.
With (b) and (c) the patient is up by the second day and weight
  bearing after 10 days.

Complications
1 Urinary tract infection (U.T.I.)
2 Hip and knee flexion contractures
3 Foot drop
4 Nerve involvement, e.g. sciatic palsy.

Precaution
With hip replacement, do not allow the patient to adduct the
  hip or flex and internally rotate the hip as dislocation can
  occur, e.g. by crossing legs when sitting.
  Check post-operative procedure with surgeon.

Fractured shaft of femur

Possible treatment
  (a) Patient put on traction for 8-10 weeks. This method is usually adopted for the younger patient as prolonged bed-rest can be detrimental for the older patient
  (b) Open reduction and internal fixation with a pin and plate or Kuntchner nail through medulla. Union occurs after 3-4 months. Exercises, especially for quadriceps contraction, are started immediately. The patient is allowed to walk non-weight bearing immediately and partially weight bearing after 4 weeks.
  (c) Cast-bracing 8-10 weeks post accident when fracture loosely united. Patient allowed to mobilise partially weight bearing ('Ling Lee' prosthesis).

Complications
1 Delayed union
2 Mal-union resulting in shortening of the femur
3 Stiff knee
4 Adhesions of quadriceps to the fracture site
5 Foot drop.

Dislocation of the hip

Congenital
Possible treatment:
  (a) Plaster immobilisation
  (b) Abduction traction
  (c) Hip replacement
  (d) Surgical reduction in infancy
  (e) Chiari procedure to deepen acetabulum when adulthood reached
  (f) Osteotomy.

Acquired
Possible treatment:
  (a) Arthroplasty
  (b) Hip spica
  (c) Traction.

Aims of treatment for hip injuries
Strengthen the lower limb
Mobilise the lower limb
Personal independence
Prevent deformities
Ensure a good walking pattern
Take proper prophylactic measures, i.e. eliminate cause of
injury, e.g. stabilise loose slip mats
Work assessment and simulation.

Functional assessment
Measure:
Range of movement at the hip
Range of movement at the knee
Quadriceps: muscle bulk and strength
Check for extension lag.

A.D.L.
Useful aids include:
Long handled shoe horn
Braces on trousers for ease in pulling up from the floor
Stocking gutter
Bath aids: bath board, seat, bath mat, bath rail
Lavatory aids, e.g. rails, raised lavatory seat
Rails on both sides of the stairs
Bed aids: blocks and boards
Helping hand
High seat chair or chair blocks.

Home visit
Check:
Height of steps: 67° of hip flexion required
Floor coverings: should be non-slip
Height of cupboards
Aids supplied
Family or other help available.

Principle of treatment
Work for stability before mobility by using resistance in the
mid-range of movement.

Activities

Early stage
Personal independence
Rug loom
Four way loom
Foot games seated: elevated noughts and crosses; dominoes
Fletcher-Wiltshire bed loom: do not encourage too wide a
    range of movement.

Middle stage
Lathe: seated on a Camden stool
Oliver bicycle
Treadle sewing machine
Treadle fret saw
A.D.L.: stair practice; walking practice; housework advice re
    sexual intercourse
Foot draughts: standing using a maxi board
Fletcher-Wiltshire bed loom.

Late stage
Benchwork for standing tolerance and balance
Quoits: standing using no sticks
Draughts: crouching
Gardening: weeding; digging; walking over rough ground
Camden cycle: can give 18° of hip extension
Cross cut sawing: for balance and weight transferance
Lathe: standing on alternate legs
Weaving: adapted with hip extension adaptation
Printing adapted: with hip extension adaptation; with hip
    flexion adaptation; with hip abduction adaptation
Housework: for stretching and crouching
Outdoor draughts: for abduction and extension of the hip
Ladder climbing
Skittles
Football
Wobble board
Work assessment and simulation.

Suggested activities for children
Games involving sitting and walking
Using linoleum with games printed on it
Riding a tricycle
Cheney walk trolley
Games to encourage abduction: balloon races with the balloon
   between the legs; maxi draughts.

Length of treatment
Young patients: 4-6 weeks
Older patients: 6-12 weeks.

Other treatment
Physiotherapy
Hydrotherapy
Remedial gym.

KNEE INJURIES AND CONDITIONS

Types
Torn meniscus
Fractured condyle of femur
Fractured tibia and fibula
Fractured fibula
Fractured tibial plateau
Fractured patella
Rheumatoid arthritis
Osteo-arthrosis
Bursitis
Ligamentous injuries.

Meniscectomy
The meniscus is removed and a pressure bandage is applied.
   Quadriceps exercises are started the following day and
   active knee mobilisation is started after 10-21 days.

Fractured tibia and fibula

Immobilisation
A walking P.O.P., from groin to metatarsals, is applied for 11

weeks, with the ankle in neutral position. The patient is
eweight bearing within 3 weeks.
After 8 weeks, the P.O.P. is often reduced to below knee.

Fractured fibula

Initial treatment
A bandage is applied and the patient walks immediately,
  because the fibula is a non-weight bearing bone.

Fractured tibial plateau

Immobilisation
The knee is aspirated and a P.O.P. is applied from groin to
  above ankle, for 6 weeks. After 10 weeks the patient is fully
  weight bearing.

Fractured patella

Stellate fracture
Immobilisation:
  (a) Walking P.O.P. for 4 weeks, groin to ankle
  (b) Patellectomy.

Transverse fracture
Initial treatment:
  (a) Fixation by screw or suture and immobilisation in P.O.P.
      from ankle to groin for 3 weeks
  (b) Patellectomy with suture of the quadriceps tendon.

Patellectomy
Immobilisation:
The operation is followed by immobilisation in P.O.P. for 3
  weeks. The patient is weight bearing after 5-6 weeks.
  Quadriceps exercises are started immediately after
  operation.

Ligamentous injuries

Torn collateral ligaments
Possible treatment:

Partial tears:
A walking P.O.P. from groin to metatarsals is applied for 3 weeks. Quadriceps exercises are started immediately.

Complete tears:
(a) A walking P.O.P. is applied from ankle to groin, for 6 weeks. Quadriceps exercises are started immediately
(b) Operation to repair tear is preferable. A P.O.P. from ankle to groin is applied and quadriceps exercises started immediately. After 2 weeks, when post-operative swelling has subsided, a new P.O.P. (walking) is applied for 4 weeks
(c) If injury not diagnosed at time of accident—e.g. if there are multiple injuries, surgical procedures to 'tighten' ligaments either lateral pivot shift operation Pes anserinus transfer.

Torn cruciate ligaments
Possible treatment
Aspiration followed by immobilisation in P.O.P. from groin to metatarsals
Quadriceps exercises are started immediately.

Precautions for knee injuries
1. Do not stretch weakened quadriceps muscles by working for flexion before extension lag has been eliminated
2 Do not work too hard for knee flexion as this can cause post operative effusion.

Complications
1 Osteoarthritic changes in the joint
2 Delayed union
3 Oedema
4 Stiff ankle
5 Prolonged extension lag.

Aims of treatment
Strengthen quadriceps muscles
Stabilise the knee joint

Mobilise the knee joint, and the ankle when necessary
Encourage a good walking pattern
Work assessment and simulation.

Principles of treatment

1 Check for extension lag; if present, do not work for flexion
2 Treat for stability before mobility—by using maximum
  resistance in the mid-range.

Activities

Early stage
To eliminate extension lag:

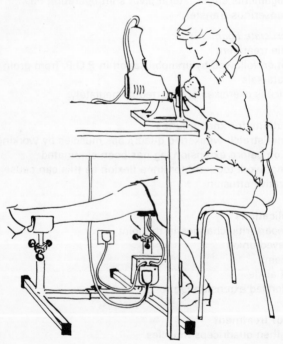

Figure 4

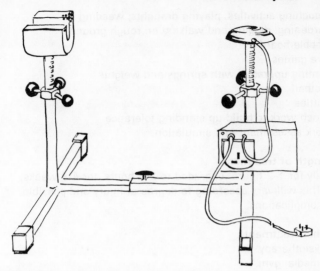

Figure 5

Lathe work: with leg slung for reciprocal quads
Bench work: with leg slung for reciprocal quads
Weaving with extension lag adaptation
Printing with extension lag adaptation
Foot games: elevated O's and X's; brick building; foot
    dominoes
Quads switch see figs 4 and 5.

Middle stage
Oliver bicycle
Lathe
Weaving with knee flexion and extension adaptations
Printing with knee flexion and extension adaptations
Stair practice using upstairs facilities
Outdoor draughts on a maxi board.

Late stage
Camden cycle: for full knee flexion
Larvic lathe: for full knee flexion

Crouching activities: playing draughts; weeding
Gardening: digging and walking on rough ground
Wobble board
Tyre games
Printing upgraded with springs and weights
Football
Skittles
Bench work to build up standing tolerance
Work assessment and simulation.

Length of treatment
Daily for 1-2 hours, upgraded to 2-4 hours, for 4-8 weeks.
  This will vary according to degree of injury and possible
  complications.

Other treatment
Physiotherapy
Remedial gym.

ANKLE INJURIES

Types
Fractured calcaneum (os calcis)
Potts fracture: varying degrees
Sprain
Ruptured achilles tendon
Fractured cuboid and navicular.

Fractured calcaneum

Possible treatment
  (a) A crepe bandage is applied for 2-3 weeks and the limb
      is kept in elevation. The patient is weight bearing after
      6-8 weeks
  (b) A walking P.O.P. is applied from metatarsals to below
      knee for 6 weeks. A pin if often inserted to hold the
      displaced calcaneum in position
  (c) Primary arthrodesis.

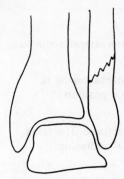

Potts fracture: First degree

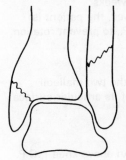

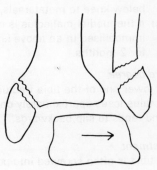

Potts fracture: Second degree

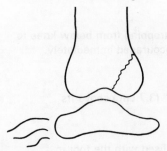

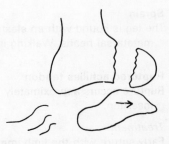

Potts fracture: Third degree

Figure 6

Potts fracture

First degree Fig. 6
This is fracture of one bone only, usually the lateral malleolus.

Treatment
A walking P.O.P. from below knee to metatarsal heads is
  applied for 4-6 weeks. The ankle is in mid-position.

Second degree
Both the medial and lateral malleoli are fractured. The talus
  slips and carries with it part of the lateral malleolus.

Treatment
  (a) Screwing of the medial malleolus and a P.O.P. from
      below knee to metatarsals, for 6-8 weeks
  (b) If the medial malleolus is not screwed, the patient is
      immobilised in an above knee P.O.P., to prevent rotation,
      for 2 months.

Third degree
The lower end of the tibia fractures plus the two malleoli
The talus loses approximately one-third of its articular surface
  and tends to slip backwards.

Treatment
The tibia is often screwed into position. An above knee P.O.P.
  is applied (to prevent rotation) for 3 months.

Sprain
The leg is bound with an elastic stropping from below knee to
  metatarsal heads. Walking is encouraged immediately.

Ruptured achilles tendon
Rupture occurs approximately 1½" (3.7 cm.) above its
  insertion.

Treatment
Early suture with the limb immobilised with the foot in
  plantarflexion and the knee slightly flexed to prevent strain
  on the tendon. Immobilisation for 4-6 weeks.

Ligamentous rupture
Rupture usually of the lateral ligament.

Immobilisation
A below knee P.O.P. (walking) is applied with the foot in slight
   eversion, for 8 weeks. Weight bearing is allowed
   immediately.

Arthrodesis
Immobilisation
Following operation, a P.O.P. is applied from below knee to
   metatarsal heads, for 3 months.

Complications
1 Osteo-arthritic changes
2 Instability due to ligamentous strain
3 Flat feet
4 Non-union
5 Pain, swelling and stiffness due to ligamentous injury
   If pain persists, often arthrodesis is performed on the ankle
6 Residual pain: especially with a fractured calcaneum
7 Lack of in and eversion.

Aims of treatment
Mobilise the ankle
Strengthen the ankle
Eliminate extension lag
Reduce oedema by elevated activities
Maintain a good walking pattern
Give gentle, rhythmical movements to reduce pain
Mobilise the knee if stiff
Work assessment and simulation.

Functional assessment
Measure:
   Plantar and dorsi-flexion
   In and eversion
   Oedema
   Knee movements.

Principle of occupational therapy
Aim for mobility followed by stability.

Activities

First stage
  (a) Treat for extension lag if present
  (b) Treat in elevation to reduce oedema
Extension lag activities:
  Weaving: with extension lag adaptation
  Printing: with extension lag adaptation
  Quads switch
  Remedial games: elevated O's and X's; elevated draughts;
  foot dominoes; all with the patient seated
Static quadriceps exercised with the leg slung under the lathe
or bench.
Activities when extension lag eliminated:
  Weaving: plantar and dorsi-flexion adaptations
  Remedial games: elevated draughts; elevated O's and X's
  Oliver bicycle
  Lathe: patient seated
  Treadle sewing machine
  Fletcher-Wiltshire bed loom: adapted for plantar and dorsi-
  flexion
  Walking practice.

Second stage
Oliver bicycle
Upright rug loom
Treadle sewing machine $\Big\}$ using wedges for in and eversion
Treadle fret-saw
Weaving: with plantar and dorsi-flexion, and in and eversion
  adaptations
Lathe work: at the front
Foot games: drawing and writing with the feet.

Third stage
Ankle rotator
Tyre games
Dancing: especially Scottish country dancing

Bench work: for standing tolerance and balance
Gardening: crouching, digging and walking on rough ground
   for in and eversion
Wobble board games
Climbing rope ladders
Weaving: in and eversion adaptations
Camden cycle
Treadle fret-saw: with in and eversion wedges
Lathe work: back for plantar and dorsi-flexion
Work assessment and simulation.

FOOT INJURIES

Types
Fractured metatarsals—including march fracture
Fractured phalanges
Flat feet
Hallux valgus (bunions)
Congenital deformities.

Fractured metatarsals
Possible treatment
   (a) Strapping for 1-2 weeks
   (b) A walking P.O.P. from below knee to metatarsal heads,
       from 6-8 weeks. The foot is immobilised in neutral
       position.

March fracture:
Occurs following a long walk or march; it is a spontaneous
   metatarsal fracture.

Possible treatment
Foot is immobilised in P.O.P. for 6 weeks.

Fractured phalanges
Possible treatment
Strapping for 1-2 weeks.

Flat feet

Causes
  (a) Failure of muscular support
  (b) Stretching of ligaments
  (c) Alteration of bone shape.

Treatment
Exercise only is usually sufficient. The correct type of footwear should be advised.

Hallux valgus (bunions)

This is a deformity of the great toe with the phalanges adducted towards the second toe. It is aggravated by tight shoes and stockings.

The skin becomes stretched and rubs against the shoe resulting in the formation of a sack of lubricant fluid.

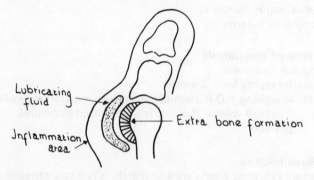

Lubricating fluid

Inflammation area

Extra bone formation

Figure 7

Possible treatment
  (a) Surgery: usually Keller's operation; the excess bone is removed and the proximal half of the proximal phalanx is exercised
  (b) Arthrodesis of the metatarso-phalangeal joint of the hallux.

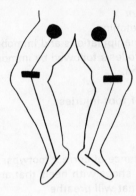

Figure 8 Equino varus

Congenital deformities

Equino varus (inversion)
There is deviation towards the mid-line with bowing of the
   legs and plantar-flexion and adduction of the forefoot, and
   inversion of the foot.

Equino valgus (eversion)
There is deviation away from the mid-line resulting in 'knock
   knees' with the foot everted, dorsiflexed and abducted.

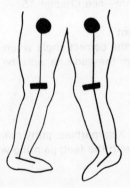

Figure 9

Possible treatment
- (a) Passive stretching
- (b) Repeated manipulations and immobilisation in P.O.P.
- (c) Triple arthrodesis followed by immobilisation in P.O.P. for 3 months.

Complications of foot injuries
Adhesions.

Precautions
Stress the importance of correct footwear:
    Lace up shoes; shoes with heels that are not too high;
    leather shoes that will breathe
    Footcare.

Aims of treatment
Encourage a good walking pattern
Encourage and strengthen arches of the foot
Encourage in and eversion, plantar and dorsi-flexion.

Joint assessment
Measure:
    In and eversion
    Plantar and dorsi-flexion.
Functional assessment—see Chapter 15.

Principle of treatment
Maintain the feet at the correct angle when treating, i.e. with the feet at 15° from the mid-line with the patellae pointing forward.

Activities
First stage
Foot games: O's and X's; marbles; putty rolling; brick building; draughts; writing with the feet; painting with the feet; foot dominoes.

Middle stage
Oliver bicycle

Treadle fret-saw
Treadle sewing machine } with in and eversion wedges
Weaving with in and eversion adaptation
Lathe: use the back of the lathe for plantar-flexion.

Late stage
Dancing: especially Scottish country dancing
Wobble board
Tyre games
Climbing rope ladders
Gardening: heavy digging
Ankle rotator
Camden cycle
Work assessment.

Other treatment
Physiotherapy
Hydrotherapy.

3 / HAND INJURIES

THE HAND

Grips
1 Plate grip
2 Cylinder grip or power grip
3 Pincer grip
4 Tripod grip
5 Ball grip
6 Span grip
7 Suitcase grip.

Measuring
Goniometer, solder wire or paper silhouette for joint
    measurement
Dynamometer for grip measurement
Grip measurement: ask the patient to grip two extended
    fingers of the therapist who has her arms crossed
Sensation testing using a pin and cotton wool.

Functional assessment
This is best done by a set functional test which could include
    some or all of the following:
    Fastening buckles
    Handling coins
    Dialling
    Fastening a watch strap
    Turning a page
    Turning off a light
    Turning door knobs
    Turning a tap

Threading a needle
Using keys
Picking up a pin
Striking a match
Fastening a safety pin
Fastening shoe laces.

Aids to daily living
Suitable aids include:
Tap turner
Ring a zip tab
Key enlarged with blocks
Cutlery handles enlarged with Rubazote
Button hook.

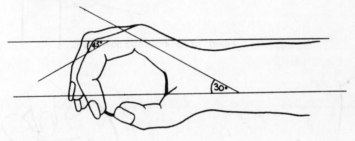

Figure 10 Position of function

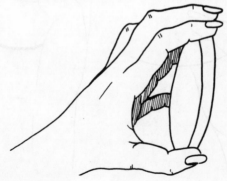

Figure 11 Span grip

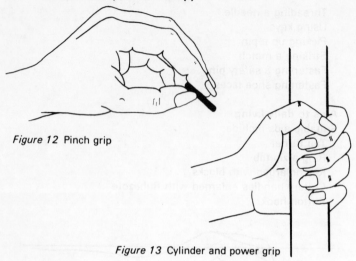

Figure 12 Pinch grip

Figure 13 Cylinder and power grip

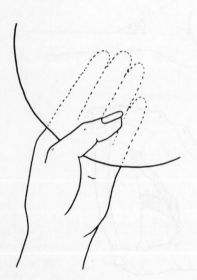

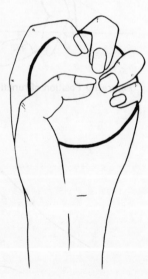

Figure 14 Plate grip

Figure 15 Ball grip

FRACTURES

Types

1 Fractured scaphoid which is immobilised for 8-32 weeks
2 Bennett's fracture which is immobilised for 6 weeks and may be internally fixed with a screw
3 Phalangeal fractures which may be displaced. Internal fixation may be used
4 Metacarpal fractures which are immobilised with a crêpe bandage for 1 week.

Complications

1 Sudeck's atrophy
2 Tendon adherence
3 Joint stiffness.

Aims of treatment

1 Work for flexion of the inter-phalangeal joints and then flexion of the metacarpo-phalangeal joints to obtain a good grip
2 Extension where necessary
3 Power grip
4 Finger dexterity.

Length of treatment

1-2 hours daily for 1-2 weeks.

Other treatment

Physiotherapy
Silastic surgery.

TENDON INJURIES

Types

1 Mallet finger
2 Boutonniere deformity
3 Trigger finger or thumb
4 Severing of the flexor tendons.

Mallet finger

This is a dropped distal phalanx due to a lesion over the middle or terminal joint.

Boutonniere deformity

This is a flexion deformity of the P.I.P. joint with hyper-extension of the D.I.P. joint. It is a lesion at the proximal phalanx involving the central slip of the tendon of extensor digitorum communis.

Trigger finger or thumb

It is a nodule on a tendon restricting movement of the finger or thumb and producing stiffness and clicking of the finger.

Sutured tendons

They are sutured and immobilised for 4-6 weeks after injury.

(a) Grafts:
   The tendons of palmaris longus, plantaris or the extensor tendons of the toes may be used to replace damaged tendons.
   The donor area should also be treated after grafting.

(b) Tendon transplants:
   Only the position of the insertion is altered, e.g. the tendon of flexor digitorum sublimis inserting on the ring finger can be transplanted to insert on the thumb, thus replacing flexor pollicis longus.

Complications

1 Stiffness of the joints
2 Oedema
3 Adhesions
4 Contractures.

Precautions

Give gentle non-resisted activities for up to 6 weeks after surgery.

Aims of treatment
1 Flexion of the I.P. joints first, followed by flexion of the M.C.P. joints
2 Strengthen grip
3 Extension of the fingers if contractures are present
4 Treat the donor graft area if necessary
5 Splintage with a double finger stall until slight voluntary movement returns.

Prognosis
Good, but rarely 100%.

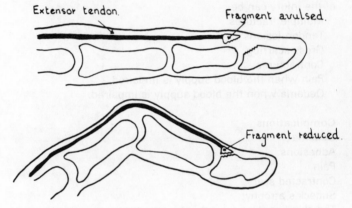

Figure 16 Mallet finger

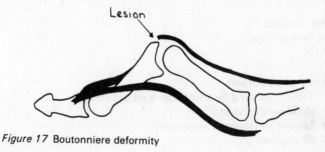

Figure 17 Boutonniere deformity

Length of treatment
Daily for 1-2 hours for 2-3 weeks.

Other treatment
Physiotherapy
Reconstructive surgery if necessary.

CRUSH INJURIES

They are mainly caused through industrial injuries. The result
of the injury can be:
   Multiple fractures
   Tendon lesions
   Gross scarring
   Contractures
   Pain when the blood supply is impaired
   Oedema when the blood supply is impaired.

Complications
Oedema
Adhesions
Pain
Contracted scars
Sudeck's atrophy:
The skin becomes smooth; shiny; cyanotic; is oedematous and
   does not pit
There is osteo-porosis of the carpus and metacarpals.

Precautions
Sensation loss
Pain.

Aims of treatment
1 Reduce oedema by using elevated activities
2 Mobilise the hand
3 Retrain sensation if necessary
4 Strengthen grip.

Length of treatment
Up to 6 months if the whole hand is involved.

Other treatments
Physiotherapy
Lively splintage if necessary
Manipulation
Surgery.

AMPUTATIONS

1 Radial:
   If the thumb is lost this is a 50% disability
2 Ulnar:
   This is less severe but the border of the hand needs toughening
3 Distal:
   This is the commonest and requires stump toughening
4 Physiological:
   Sensation retraining and re-education of grip are required.

Precautions
Pain
Hypersensitivity of the stump
New skin which is tender and susceptible to injury.

Aims of treatment
1 Boost morale as a large psychological factor is involved
2 Toughen the stump
3 Densensitise the stump
4 Reduce the oedema by using elevated activities
5 Mobilise the hand
6 Re-education of nerve function and manual dexterity
7 Splintage:
   In the form of a cuff if the whole hand has been amputated
   In the form of a built up stump if the thumb has been amputated.

Length of treatment
2 hours daily for 2-3 weeks.

Activities
Percussion of the stump.

Other treatments
Reconstructive surgery, e.g. pollicisation.
Methods of reconstruction include:
1 Lengthening of the thumb flap by a local flap and bone graft
2 Pollicisation of one of the fingers
3 Reconstruction by tube pedicle and bone graft
4 Transfer of a toe.
Samll functional prosthesis where necessary.

DUPUYTREN'S CONTRACTURE

It is an affectation of the palmar fascia causing a flexion
contracture of the M.P. joints and the proximal I.P. joints, and
extension of the distal I.P. joints. It appears as a small nodule
on the palmar surface of the hand and usually occurs in the
ring and little fingers. It can be bilateral and may affect the
feet. It can take 3 months to 20 years from the primary nodule
to the full contracture.

Complication
Recurrence.

Aims of treatment
1 Increase flexion
2 Increase extension
3 Function of the hand related to the job.

Prognosis
Early surgery has good results otherwise recurrence of the
contracture may occur.

Length of treatment
Daily for at least 1 hour for 2 weeks.

Other treatment
Physiotherapy
Serial splintage: provided by O.T.s or physiotherapists
Stretch splintage: provided by O.T.s or physiotherapists.

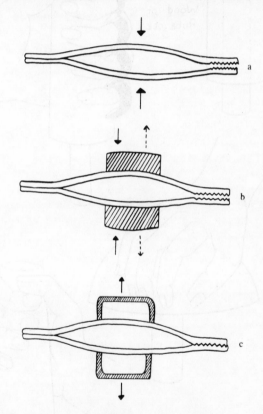

Figure 18 Tweezers: (a) Unadapted
(b) Adapted for passive extension
(c) Adapted for active extension

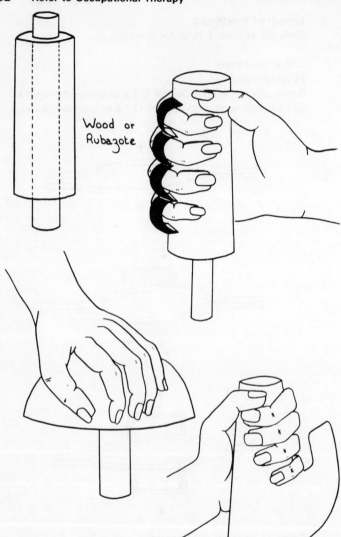

Wood or Rubazote

Figure 19 Adaptations to plane handles

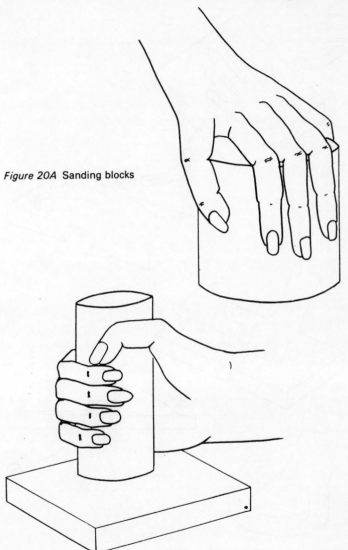

Figure 20A Sanding blocks

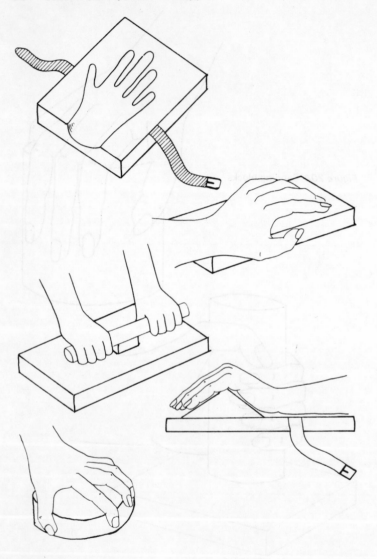

Figure 20B Sanding blocks

ACTIVITIES USED IN THE TREATMENT OF THE HAND

Activities	I.P. flex	M.P. flex	Active ext	Passive ext	Gross grip	Opposition	Dexterity	Sensation	Elevation
LARGE:									
Solitaire		✓				✓			✓
Draughts	✓			✓		✓			
Peggotty				✓		✓			
Span game	✓			✓		✓			✓
Dominoes	✓			✓				✓	
SMALL:									
Solitaire		✓				✓	✓		
Draughts		✓				✓	✓		
Peggotty		✓				✓	✓	✓	
Dominoes	✓	✓				✓	✓		
Cat's cradle	✓	✓	✓			✓			
Puff football and water syphon	✓	✓			✓	✓			
Puff football and water syphon using pinch grip		✓				✓			
Table tennis	✓	✓		✓ INDEX	✓	✓			
Bagatelle and ping-pong-flicking	✓		✓						
With stick or spring	✓					✓			
Cards		✓		✓			✓		
Origami		✓		✓			✓		
Scissors			✓	✓			✓		
Pottery	✓	✓	✓	✓	✓	✓	✓	✓	✓
Stool seating	✓	✓				✓	✓		✓
Basketry		✓		✓					✓
Cooking:									
Pastry mixing		✓				✓		✓	
Pastry rolling			✓						
Creaming and beating	✓	✓			✓				
Peeling	✓	✓							
Making bread	✓	✓							
Chopping herbs		✓				✓			

Activities	I.P. flex	M.P. flex	Active ext	Passive ext	Gross grip	Opposition	Dexterity	Sensation	Elevation
PRINTING:									
F.E.P.S. roller	✓	✓			✓				
F.E.P.S. wheel	✓					✓			
Bell rope	✓	✓			✓			✓	✓
Spade handle	✓								✓
Cotton reel	✓	✓							✓
Extension board				✓					
Unadapted		✓			✓				
Picking up paper		✓				✓	✓		✓
Composing	✓	✓				✓	✓		
Composing with									
tweezers		✓				✓	✓		
with padded									
tweezers				✓		✓	✓		
loop handled									
tweezers			✓			✓	✓		
WEAVING:									
Unadapted		✓				✓	✓		
Adapted (see									
printing)									
WOODWORK:									
Sawing			index		✓	✓			✓
Planing	✓	✓			✓	✓			
(see diagrams									
of adapted									
handles)									
Screwing	✓	✓	✓		✓	✓			✓
Sanding									
(N.B. adapted									
blocks)								✓	
Screwing with ratchet	✓	✓			✓				
Hammer/mallet	✓	✓			✓				
Macramé (cord									
knotting)	✓	✓			✓	✓	✓	✓	
PAINTING:									
Finger			✓	✓			✓		
Small brush		✓				✓	✓		
Large brush		✓			✓	✓			
Pea game		✓	✓			✓			

Activities	I.P. flex	M.P. flex	Active ext	Passive ext	Gross grip	Opposition	Dexterity	Sensation	Elevation
Lentils on the hand							✓	✓	
Penny on the hand			✓				✓		
GARDENING:									
Weeding			✓		✓	✓		✓	
Trowel	✓	✓			✓	✓			
Pruning	✓			✓	✓	✓			
Pricking out seedlings		✓				✓	✓	✓	
Wrought iron work		✓		✓	✓				
Rug weaving									
Tufts								✓	✓
Beating		✓		✓					
ARCHERY:									
String hand	✓								

4 / BACK INJURIES

BACK INJURIES

Types
Prolapsed intervertebral disc
Ankylosing spondylitis
Cervical spondylitis
Osteo-arthrosis of the spine
Fracture or dislocation.

Signs and symptoms
Pain
Weakness in limbs
Paraesthesia
Restricted movement
Apprehension and fear of further injury.

Complications
1 Paralysis
2 Sciatica.

Precautions
1 No flexion until later stages
2 Teach lifting with straight back
3 No heavy work until later stages
4 Do not overwork patient or symptoms may be exacerbated
5 Advice re sitting position.

Specific policies
To be checked with doctor
1 Extension followed by slight flexion in last stage

2 Flexion and rotation immediately
3 Isometric flexion only.

Aims of treatment

1 Strengthen back and limbs if necessary
2 Alleviate pain
3 Prophylactic measures.

Functional assessment

Reassurance must be given as to condition and possible
further pain
Test sitting and standing tolerance
Check lifting technique: keep the back straight
Verbal assessment of attitude.

A.D.L.

Chair: check height and back support
Dressing routine including labour saving techniques
Sitting for housework
Firm bed or fracture boards
Long handled tools where necessary.

Activities

For extension
Rug loom
Printing: overhead bar
Woodwork: high bench
Games, elevated
Stool seating: high
Archery
Window cleaning: high
Painting: high.

For slight flexion
Polishing
Sanding
Hoeing
Raking

Generally working at lower levels.

For flexion and rotation
Position work to obtain the movement in:
    Games
    Printing
    Industrial work
    Bench work
    Large assembly work.

For isometric flexion
Oliver bicycle: mid-position with increased resistance
Bench work at correct height adjustment.

Toughening activities
Cross-cut sawing
Lathe work: standing on alternate legs
Gardening: hedge clipping; digging; rolling; lawn mowing
Archery: to encourage a good posture.

Relief of pain
Teach the patient to stand with back flat against the wall with
    feet 12 to 18 inches in front of him when he has acute
    pain. This eases the intensity.

Length of treatment
One hour daily increasing time to a full day; 6 weeks
    maximum.

Other treatment
Physiotherapy
Surgery
Drugs.

5 / NERVE LESIONS

NERVE LESIONS

There are three main types of lesion which are classified according to the amount of damage sustained.

Neuropraxia
Damage to the nerve by pressure. Recovery is usually within 6 weeks.

Axonotmesis
The axon is severed, but the sheath remains intact. It is a rare injury resulting from stretching. Recovery is good.

Neurotmesis
Severance of the axon, cylinder and sheath. Recovery is rarely complete as only a small proportion of axons return to their original end organs.

The rate of growth is approximately 1mm a day. The amount of recovery can be estimated by Tinel's sign, which is pain over the growth cone.

BRACHIAL PLEXUS

Cause of injury
Blow or fall on shoulder.

Types of injury
1 Direct—stab wound pressure
2 Traction—in continuity avulsion.

Signs and symptoms
Flail upper limb and weak shoulder
Extensive sensation loss.

Precautions and complications
Brachial plexus or hemiplegic sling to prevent further damage
    to shoulder and subluxation
Desensitisation
Do not over stretch weak muscle
Frozen shoulder
Circulation poor in cold weather.

Aims of treatment
Personal independence
Sensation training
Maintain range of movement
Splintage e.g. flail arm splint with terminal appliances used as
    prostheses
Re-educate function as it returns.

O.T. approach
Depression expected if long wait for recovery
With the permission of the doctor realistic information should
    be given of the future.

A.D.L.
One-handed methods
May need writing practice
Two handed activities using splint and terminal appliances in
    bi-lateral pattern.

Activities
In O.B. help arm
Bilateral activities
Stereognosis
Games
Assisted printing
Polishing

Planing with hand strapped
Oliver bicycle, with hand strapped and an elbow support for
   vibrations
Work assessment
Re-training with splint appliances.

When recovery
Weaving
Stool seating
Rug loom
Printing with S.H.E.A.F.E.; overhead bar
Games in elevation
Cooking
Gardening
Progress to finer activities as recovery occurs
Work assessment.

Prognosis
After 2 years, if there is no recovery then possible amputation
  or surgical exploration; repair of some nerves by nerve
  grafts to give some return of function.

Length of treatment
When first referred, daily for 4 weeks, then intermittently from
   6 months to 3 years.

Other treatments
Physiotherapy
Tendon transfers
Joint fusion in functional position e.g. wrist.

DELTOID PALSY

Cause of injury
Blow on shoulder
Stretching shoulder
Stretching arm.

Signs and symptoms
No true abduction.

Precautions and complications
Frozen shoulder.

Aims of treatment
Teach trick movement:
> This is used to get the shoulder into abduction, enabling the joint to remain mobile, otherwise a frozen shoulder will result
> External rotation: infra spinatus; teres minor
> Flexion: biceps (long head)
> Movement finished by: pectoralis major; serratus anterior
> This may be done in conjunction with the physiotherapist and the patient can be discharged continuing with the trick movement until recovery occurs.

Maintain range
Specific treatment when recovery occurs.

Activities
Before recovery
If the trick movement is not taught, specific treatment given only to facilitate motor return.
Printing: overhead bar
Archery
Elevated draughts
Gardening
Weaving
Painting
Stool seating
Window cleaning.

As recovery occurs
Printing S.H.E.A.F.E.; spade handle to side, pulling down then up; paper at side
Bilateral wire twister
Rug loom.

Length of treatment
6 weeks after the nerve begins to recover.

Other treatment
Physiotherapy.

RADIAL NERVE LESION

Cause of injury
Fractured shaft of humerus
Crutch palsy
'Saturday night palsy', i.e. patient falling asleep with the arm
over the back of a chair.

Signs and symptoms
Drop wrist
Lack of finger extension
Sensation loss
If the level of the injury is high, triceps is affected resulting in
weak elbow extension.

Complication
Capsulitis.

Precautions
Prevent over-stretching of weak muscles.

Aims of treatment
1 Maintain range and power in the whole upper limb
2 Treat for wrist and finger extension as recovery occurs
3 Teach the trick movement of flexing the wrist to extend the
fingers. This can be used until some innervation takes place
4 Strengthen grip
5 Splintage to provide a position of function and to prevent
stretching of weak muscles. It should take the form of a
lively cock-up splint.

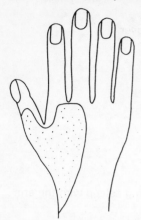

Figure 21 Sensory distribution
of radial nerve

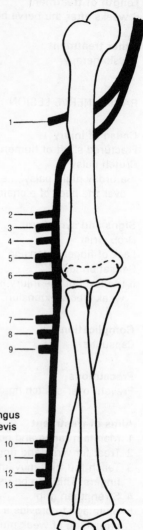

Distribution of radial nerve

Figure 22   1 – Triceps
2 – Brachio-radialis
3 – Extensor carpi radialis longus
4 – Extensor carpi radialis brevis
5 – Supinator
6 – Anconeus
7 – Extensor digitorum
8 – Extensor digiti minimi
9 – Extensor carpi ulnaris
10 – Abductor pollicis longus
11 – Extensor pollicis longus
12 – Extensor pollicis brevis
13 – Extensor indicis

Activities
Before recovery
Weaving
Stool-seating
Painting
Elevated draughts.

As recovery occurs
Large dominoes
Cat's cradle
Flicking a ping pong ball
Large scissors: using them to cut paper, material etc.
Coil pottery
Pastry rolling
Finger painting
Beating the warp upwards on a rug loom
Printing adapted with: F.E.P.S. using the large wheel; or roller
    handle
Weaving adapted with: F.E.P.S. using the large wheel; or roller
    handle.

Length of treatment
Initially when the patient is referred: daily for 2-3 weeks
Once innervation returns a further treatment period is
    required: daily for 4 weeks.

Other treatment
Physiotherapy.

MEDIAN NERVE

Cause of injury
Severance at wrist.

Signs and symptoms
Monkey hand: loss of ability to oppose thumb
Hyper extension deformity at M.P. joints of the index and
    middle fingers
Sensory loss.

Precaution

De-sensitised skin: warn the patient about smoking and
  burning.

Aims of treatment

Maintain range and power in the whole of the upper limb
Treat for opposition and dexterity as recovery occurs
Strengthen grip
Splintage to provise a functional hand: opponens splint with
  'T' bar to prevent contracture.

Activities

Sensation training
Stereognosis: texture dominoes
Wide bilateral movements: weaving; stool seating.

Specific activities as recovery occurs
Movements for opposition to all fingers and dexterity:
  Peggotty
  Composing

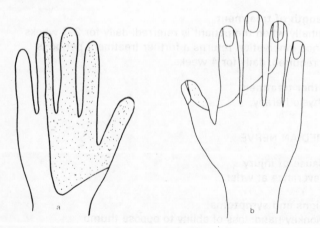

Figure 23 Sensory distribution of median nerve
          (a) Palmar view
          (b) Dorsal view

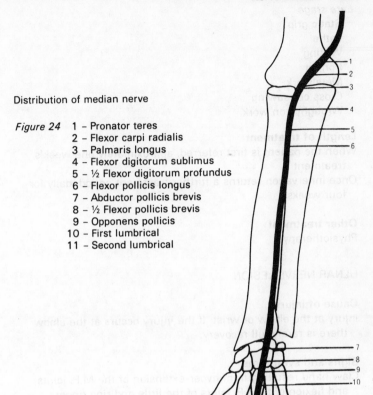

Distribution of median nerve

Figure 24   1 – Pronator teres
2 – Flexor carpi radialis
3 – Palmaris longus
4 – Flexor digitorum sublimus
5 – ½ Flexor digitorum profundus
6 – Flexor pollicis longus
7 – Abductor pollicis brevis
8 – ½ Flexor pollicis brevis
9 – Opponens pollicis
10 – First lumbrical
11 – Second lumbrical

Industrial work
Origami
Finger puppets
Scissors
Weaving with a small shuttle
Pastry making
Basketry
Cord knotting.

Late stage
- Static grip
- Lathe
- Writing
- Ironing
- Metalwork
- Cross cut sawing
- Wrought iron work.

Length of treatment
When the patient is first referred, approximately one week's treatment

Once innervation returns a further treatment period, daily for four weeks.

Other treatment
Physiotherapy.

ULNAR NERVE LESION

Cause of injury
Injury at the elbow or wrist. If the injury occurs at the elbow there is rarely full recovery.

Signs and symptoms
Claw hand resulting from hyper-extension of the M.P. joints and flexion of the I.P. joints of the little and ring fingers. When the injury occurs at the elbow the deformity is less severe at first, owing to paralysis of half of flexor digitorum profundus. As recovery occurs the claw deformity increases because innervation returns to flexor digitorum profundus, and the deformity decreases when the innervation returns to the intrinsic muscles of the hand

Sensory loss.

Precautions
Sensory loss: warn the patient about dangers of rubbing or burning the skin.

Aims of treatment

1 Maintain range of movement in the whole upper limb
2 Maintain strength in the upper limb
3 Treat for finger dexterity as recovery occurs
4 Strengthen grip
5 Splintage to provide a functional hand and prevent deformity at the M.P. joints, i.e. 'knuckle duster' splint.

Activities

Before recovery

Sensation re-training
Stereognosis: texture dominoes
Activities providing wide bilateral movements.

As recovery occurs the specific activities include

Cabinet scraping
Sharpening plane blades
Dried peas game

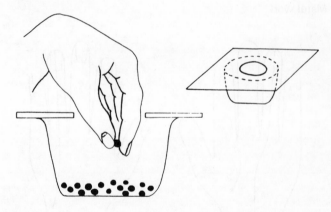

Figure 25 The hole must be small enough to allow entry of the digits only

Using dressmaker's scissors
Large draughts
Printing adapted with large F.E.P.S. wheel; or cotton reel

Weaving adapted with large F.E.P.S. wheel
Cord knotting (macrame)
Screw driving
Hammering and malleting
Using a chisel
Typing
Playing a piano or guitar
Peggotty
Composing
Pastry mixing.
These activities encourage finger dexterity, abduction of digits
   and flexion of little finger, ring finger and M.P. joints.

Late stage
Activities to produce static grip:
Lathe work
Writing
Ironing
Metal work

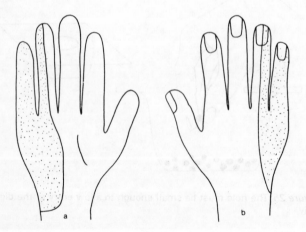

Figure 26 Sensory distribution of ulnar nerve
         (a) Palmar view
         (b) Dorsal view

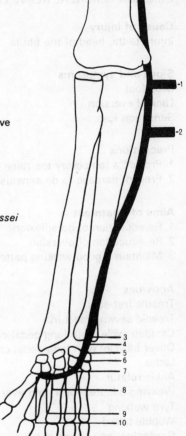

Figure 27 Distribution of ulnar nerve
1 – Flexor carpi ulnaris
2 – Flexor digitorum profundus
3 – Palmaris brevis
4 – Abductor
5 – Opponens } *digiti minimi*
6 – Flexor)
7 – Third and fourth lumbricals
8 – First palmar and dorsal interossei
9 – ½ Flexor pollicis brevis
10 – Adductor pollicis

Cross-cut sawing
Wrought iron work.

Length of treatment
When the patient is initially referred: one week's treatment
Once innervation returns a further treatment period daily for
    four weeks is required.

Other treatment
Physiotherapy.

COMMON PERONEAL NERVE LESION

Cause of injury
Injury to the head of the fibula.

Signs and symptoms
Drop foot
Lack of eversion
Sensation loss.

Precautions
1 Provide a temporary toe raise to prevent tripping
2 Prevent damage to de-sensitised skin of the feet.

Aims of treatment
1 Re-education of dorsiflexion
2 Re-education of eversion
3 Maintain a good walking pattern.

Activities
Treadle fret-saw
Treadle sewing machine
Camden cycle: with long pedal crank
Oliver bicycle: with long pedal crank
Lathe
Ankle rotator
Weaving adapted for in and eversion, plantar and dorsiflexion
Tyre walking
Wobble board
Gardening: on uneven ground
Use of wedges on foot plates.

Length of treatment
When innervation returns: 2 hours daily for 3-4 weeks.

Other treatment
Physiotherapy.

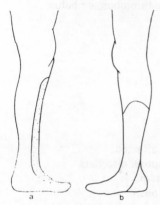

Figure 28 Posterior view of patient's feet on the foot plate
    (a) Normal position
    (b) Eversion wedge
    (c) Inversion wedge

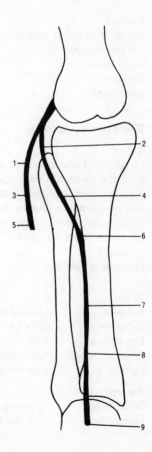

Figure 29 Sensory distribution
    of common peroneal nerve
    (a) Medial view
    (b) Lateral view

Figure 30 Distribution of
    common peroneal nerve
    1 – Superficial branch
    2 – Deep branch
    3 – Peroneus longus
    4 – Tibialis anterior
    5 – Peroneus brevis
    6 – Extensor digitorum longus
    7 – Extensor hallucis longus
    8 – Peroneus tertius
    9 – Extensor digitorum brevis

6 / HEMIPLEGIA

HEMIPLEGIA

Causes
Cerebral vascular accident (C.V.A.): thrombus; embolus; haemorrhage
Head injury
Tumour
Congenital.

Signs and symptoms

Motor
Paralysis of one side of the body
If on the dominant side: speech is affected
If on the non-dominant side: perceptual disorders
Spastic paralysis of arm: flexor spasm
Spastic paralysis of leg: extensor spasm
Paralysis starts flaccid for 2 weeks; the majority then become spastic
Balance is affected

Speech
Aphasia   : Lack of ability to talk
Dysphasia   : difficulty in enunciation
Dysarthria   : difficulty with articulation
Perseveration : repetition of meaningless words and phrases
Echolalia   : repeating what has been said.

Perceptual
Body image   : ignoring affected side
Hemianopia   : half visual field

Receptive dysphasia	: comprehension difficulties
Diplopia	: double vision
Disorientation	
Apraxia	: inability to carry out the action although the instruction is understood.

Psychological
Frustration
Depression
Apathy
Lethargy
Slowing of mental processes
Emotional lability.

Precautions
1 With a C.V.A. do not over work in case of recurrence
2 Overstretching of spastic muscles increases spasticity
3 Damage to paralysed side in a wheelchair or when walking through doors
4 Overtiring can produce perseveration.

Aims of treatment
1 Raise morale and help adjustment to disability
2 Personal independence
3 Prevent contractures
4 Obtain maximum return of function. If no return, concentrate on unaffected side
5 Resettlement.

A.D.L.
One handed aids as required
Dressing: affected side first
Bath: sound side in first, if necessary protect the back from the taps
Hemiplegic sling
Temporary toe raise with bandage held in hand
Toe raise splint
Night resting splint.

Home visit

Points to look for should include:

  Kitchen: one handed equipment; trolley; non-slip surfaces

  Rails in bathroom and lavatory

  Handrails on stairs

  Loose mats

  Family or other help available.

Activities

Sanding in a sprung sling

Polishing in a sprung sling

Oliver bicycle: to encourage a good walking pattern

Printing: unadapted

Planing: hand stropped to plane

Bilateral sawing

Wire twister: bilateral handle using a mitten glove

Housework

Lathe: seated, propelling the lathe with another person

Perceptual activities:

  Post-box

  Draughts

  Peggotty

  Chinese chequers

  Connect

Writing practice.

Prognosis

Generally poor

If there is no recovery within 6 weeks, little should be
  expected

If the cause is a Road Traffic Accident (R.T.A.) the prognosis is
  better and there is gradual recovery over a longer period of
  time.

Length of treatment

Patient should be discharged after independance has been
  achieved, i.e. 6 weeks

Follow up service or day centre reduces the length of
  treatment.

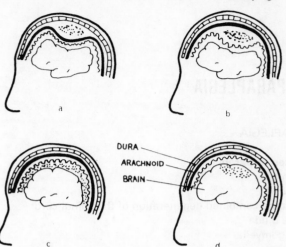

Figure 31 Diagrams to show types of intracranial haemorrhage
        (a) Extra-dural haemorrhage
        (b) Sub-dural haemorrhage
        (c) Sub-arachnoid haemorrhage
        (d) Intracerebral haemorrhage

Other treatments
Physiotherapy
Hydrotherapy
Speech therapy
Remedial gym
Social worker
Orthoptist.

Community services
Community nurse
Meals on wheels
Social Service Department.

7 / PARAPLEGIA

PARAPLEGIA

Causes of paraplegia
Trauma
Infection
Subacute combined degeneration of the spinal cord
Spina bifida
Syringomyelia
Transverse myelitis
Anterior poliomyelitis
Multiple sclerosis
Cerebral palsy.

Levels of injury

Above C5
Usually respiratory involvement leading to death.

C5 level
Full innervation to:
  Trapezius
  Teres minor
  Sternomastoid
  Upper cervical muscles.
Partial innervation to:
  Deltoid
  Infraspinatus
  Supraspinatus
  Rhomboids
  Biceps.
Able to:

Rotate neck
Move scapuli a little
Weakly abduct, flex and extend the shoulder
Flex the elbow.
Cannot:
Roll over
Sit
Use hands unaided, i.e. needs aid for feeding and washing.
Endurance is low due to reduced respiratory reserve.

C6 level
Full innervation to:
Biceps
Rotators of the shoulder
Brachioradialis.
Partial innervation to:
Latissimus dorsi
Pectoralis major
Serratus anterior
Wrist flexors and extensors
Triceps.
Able to:
Adduct the shoulder
Grasp weakly using the wrist
Assist in bed rolling
Propel a wheelchair fitted with capstan wheels on a smooth
surface
Shave with an electric razor if the plug is inserted for them
Type if helped with insertion of the paper.
Cannot:
Get into a chair
Get on to the lavatory.

C7 level
Full innervation to:
All shoulder muscles.
Partial innervation to:
Triceps
Flexors and extensors of the fingers.

Able to:
    Grasp and release
    Roll in bed
    Sit up
    Be independent in a wheelchair except over rough ground
    Dress upper half
    Manage the lavatory if rails are provided
    Drive if vehicle has hand controls and power assisted steering
    Walk if latissimus dorsi is strong enough
    Work sitting, e.g. book-keeping or typing.

T1 level

Full innervation to:
    Upper limb.
Able to:
    Move in bed
    Transfer
    Walk with braces or crutches
    Do any type of sedentary work
    Drive but has difficulty placing chair in car as the trunk is unstable.
Cannot:
    Stabilise the trunk because the upper limb fixators are not 100% efficient.
Respiratory reserves are still not completely functioning to their full capacity.

T5 level

Blood pressure is controlled
Circulation functions are normally below this level.

T6 level

Full innervation of:
    Upper costal muscles
    Upper back muscles.
Able to:
    Walk with a brace
    Pull up to the walking position
    Climb low stairs

Lift because the trunk is stable and so they can lift the wheelchair into the car.

Cannot:

Stop himself falling, so swing to gait has to be watched, to make sure they do not swing too far forward.

T12 level

Full:

Abdominal power

Pelvic control.

Able to:

Manage steps of normal height (8", 20 cm) and therefore work access is no problem

Manage without a chair during the day.

Signs and symptoms

Loss of function and muscle wasting below level of injury

Loss of sensation below level of injury

Incontinence

Psychological overlay.

Complications

Urinary tract infections (U.T.I.)

Pressure sores.

Precautions

Contractures of the flexor muscles

Poor skin condition

Poor circulation: pooling of the blood in the feet may lead to loss of consciousness on standing.

Aims of treatment

1 Personal independence
2 Wheelchair assessment
  Walking aid assessment
3 Work assessment and resettlement
4 Strengthen upper limb and back muscles
5 Maintain residual function
6 Build up morale

7 Prevent muscle contractures
8 Reinforce skin care
9 During bed rest start assessment and investigations into home and work situations as both may take a long while to adapt or change.

Functional assessment
1 Assess patient's residual function, e.g. standing ability; balance; ability to do press-ups.
2 A.D.L.
  Aids e.g.
    Helping hand
    Bags on wheelchair
    Long handled shoe horn
  Clothing:
    Two piece dresses
    Short coats for use in a wheelchair
    Slacks with a zip up both sides
    Raglan sleeves
    Wrap over skirts
    Clothes a size larger than the person would normally take
    Elastic topped stockings; not too tight
  Stretch socks to avoid abrasive wrinkles
    Pants with a side fastening with loose elastic round the waist.

Dressing method
1 Dress lower half on the bed where spasm will not result in a fall
2 Sit with the legs straight in front of them
3 Pull up one leg and put foot into pants
4 Pull up to mid calf
5 Put second leg into pants
6 Work up over knees
7 Lie down and pull up over buttocks rolling from side to side.
Adaptations to clothing:
  Zip on inside trouser leg seam for easy dressing and emptying of urinary bag.

Ensure the patient does not sit on wrinkled clothes in the wheelchair.

3 Home visit; points to be noted should include:
   Height of switches
   Loose mats
   Width of doors
   Floor surfaces should be non slip
   Odd steps in passages and steps up to the door
   Bedroom should be downstairs
   Position of bathroom
   Type of building structure if electrical hoists are required
   Height of kitchen work surfaces
   Width of passageways.

4 Wheelchair assessment
   May also need:
   Sheepskin
   Ripple cushion
   Paraplegic cushion
   Desk arms
   Leg straps
   Tray
   Capstan wheels
   Transference to chair; to the lavatory; to the bed
   Assess if a hoist is necessary.

Methods of transferring

Wheelchair to bed
   (a) Bed approximately same height as wheelchair
   (b) Place wheelchair at right angles to the bed with front wheels a few inches from the side
   (c) Lock brakes
   (d) Lift one leg then the other onto the bed
   (e) Bring wheelchair as close as possible to the bed
   (f) By pushing on the arm and then the mattress, wriggle on to the bed, keeping head and trunk forward.

2 Sideways
   (a) Place the wheelchair close to the side of the bed, facing the head end

   (b) Slide forward moving hips towards the bed but with knees turned away

   (c) Put near hand on the bed and the other on the armrest

   (d) Push up and swing the body onto the bed.

Wheelchair to lavatory

1 Forward

   (a) Front wheels should be against the front of the lavatory, foot rests up and brakes locked

   (b) With the knees apart, slide forward onto the lavatory

   (c) To get off the lavatory, slide backwards.

   If the lavatory is too low for this, a raised toilet seat should be used.

2 Sideways: used if the bathroom is wide enough

   (a) With wheels against the side of the toilet, remove the appropriate arm rest

   (b) Make sure the brakes are locked and transfer either by several push ups or by wriggling across.

Wheelchair to another chair

Sliding

   (a) Right front wheel should be against the left front leg of the chair

   (b) The right knee should be as close as possible to the right front leg of the chair

   (c) Brakes should be locked and the footrests up

   (d) Left hand should be on the arm rest and right hand on the seat of the chair

   (e) Push up and slide from the wheelchair to the chair.

Aids for the paraplegic housewife

1 The whole kitchen should be designed for her needs including correct working heights with pull out surfaces to extend over the arms of her wheelchair

2 The sink should be at the correct height so that the knees fit underneath. Can be kidney shaped to allow her to get nearer in a wheelchair or one bowl on top of another upside down makes work easier

3 Split level ovens with the hotplates viewed in a tilted mirror

allows housewife to see inside the saucepan. To prevent the mirror from steaming up wipe with a solution of one part methylated spirits to one part glycerine

4 Wheelchair tray on which to carry hot dishes to prevent injuries to the legs due to loss of sensation

5 Rotating cupboard to allow ingredients to be obtained with ease

6 Power points at a suitable height

7 Long handled dustpan and brush

8 Windows should preferably be of the sliding type as these can be opened more easily from a wheelchair

9 Blinds are easier to operate than curtains.

Activities

Rug loom

Wire twisting machine

Bench work

Elevated sawing simulator

Stool seating

Archery

Housework: cooking; cleaning; shopping; laying table; bed making

Gardening: wheelchair garden; cutting hedges; flower arranging; greenhouse gardening

Printing using a mirror to see the work

Remedial games: low on the ground for sitting balance

Elevated sanding

Elevated draughts

Darts

Quoits

Weaving

Metal work

Swimming: with the men catheterised and the women padded; bowels should be evacuated before swimming

Ball throwing

Standing: to prevent contractures; to improve circulation

Wheelchair mobility: obstacle race; slopes and kerbs; general manoeuverability.

Morale

1 Encourage the patient to join clubs. Mixed clubs for the fit and chairbound may be of particular use
2 Give advice on marriage if the patient shows concern about this. Check with the doctor first on the advisability of marriage and pregnancy, remembering the possibility of the hereditary factor of the disease and the complications of pregnancy
3 Discussion in groups about the problems encountered.

Work assessment and rehabilitation

It may take the form of:
    Retraining
    Resettlement
    Special schools and accommodation
    Sheltered workshop.

Long term recreation

These may include:
    Archery
    Table tennis
    Chess
    Card games
    Darts
    Horse riding

Length of treatment

Daily to maximum independence for 8 weeks to 3 months.

Other treatments

Nursing care
Physiotherapy
Hydrotherapy
Remedial gym.

Paraparesis

Activities for the lower limbs:
    Oliver bicycle
    Lathe
    Treadle fret saw
    Treadle sewing machine.

ACTIVITIES CHART

	C5	C6	C7	T1	T6	T12
Eating						
Dressing						
Toileting						
Bed independence						
Wheelchair independent transfer						
Walking and able to stand alone						
Housebound work						
Outside job						
Private car independence						
Use of public transport						
Attendant to lift						
Attendant to assist						
	H LLB, PB SA	H	H	H LLB, PB, SA	LLB PB. SA	LLB PB.SA	PB.

KEY   H = Hand splint   PB = pelvic band
         LLB = long leg brace   SA = spinal attachment

8 / HEAD INJURIES

HEAD INJURIES

Causes

Trauma
R.T.A.
Prenatal or neonatal damage.

Neoplasms (tumour)
Glioma: from cerebral and cerebellar cells
Meningeoma: from arachnoid matter
Acoustic neuroma: from VIIIth cranial nerve
Blood vessel neuroma: within cranial vessels
Pituitary tumours
Metastic tumours: secondary growths.

Brain damage

Concussion
Widespread paralysis of the functions of the brain with a
   tendency to spontaneous recovery.

Contusion
Oedema and capillary haemorrhage within the brain
   accompanied by unconsciousness:
   (a) coma, which may increase until death. The longer the
       coma, the more severe the damage.
   (b) stupor: a partial consciousness which may last for years.

Laceration
A severe contusion which results in a visual breach in the
   brain substance. There is never full recovery.

Compression
Patient usually lives for only 1-2 weeks.

Phases of consciousness

1 Deep coma. Patient does not move or respond at all. At this stage the patient is often referred to O.T.
2 Withdrawal from pain: this is a sign of withdrawal from coma
3 Spontaneous movement in bed
   Patient able to swallow fluids
4 Patient will respond to his name
5 Patient will answer simple questions and obey simple commands
   Can be irritable, noisy, abusive and negativistic
6 Patient is more co-operative. May show confusion, impaired memory, emotional instability
7 Fully conscious.

Possible signs and symptoms

Motor
Ataxia
Paralysis: hemiplegia; monoplegia; quadraplegia
Inco-ordination
Poor balance
Giddiness
Headaches
Low fatigue level
Cerebral irritation: epilepsy.

Perceptual
Hemianopia: half visual field
Diplopia: double vision
Disturbance of body image
Colour and number indiscrimination
Apraxia: inability to carry out the action although the instruction is understood
Disorientation
Perceptive dysphasia: difficulty in comprehension

Noise and light intolerance

Speech
Aphasia: inability to talk
Dysphasia: difficulty in ennunciation
Dysarthria: difficulty with articulation
Perseveration: repetition of meaningless words and phrases
Echolalia: repetition of what has been said.

Psychological
Personality changes:
Irritability ⟷ apathy
Violence and anxiety ⟷ timidity
Emotional lability ⟷ emotional blunting
Depression ⟷ euphoria
Lethargy ⟷ hypomania
Slowing of mental processes
Retardation of intelligence
Frustration
Inability to concentrate
Inability to remember recent instructions
Amnesia: retro-grade; antero-grade.

Precautions
The co-operation of the patient is of prime importance,
    therefore the patient should not be overworked.
The patient should always be treated as an adult in spite of
    his disability.

Aims of treatment
1 Assessment: physical and psychological
2 Increase personal independence
3 Build up general tolerance
4 Improve morale, and encourage socialisation
5 Specific treatment for individual symptoms
6 Preparation for resettlement at work and home
7 Involve the family in the treatment programme.

Activities

Assessment

Before the treatment programme can be planned, the patient's physical and psychological capabilities must be assessed. Therefore the patient's previous personality must be ascertained from close family or friends.

A comprehensive range of activities should be chosen, and can include the following:

Upper limb function test (see appendix)

Oliver bicycle:

Sitting balance and tolerance

Muscle power of lower limb

Co-ordination of upper and lower limb

Hand—eye co-ordination

Work tolerance

Noise tolerance

Tolerance of moving machinery

Benchwork:

Upper limb strength and function

Manual dexterity

Work tolerance

Ability to follow written and verbal instructions

Mobility

Standing tolerance and balance

Posture

Responsibility

Printing:

Upper limb co-ordination

Concentration

Level of frustration

Finger dexterity

Visio-spatial ability

Initiative

Accuracy

Industrial work:

Sociability

Number and colour recognition

Speed

Memory
Concentration
Tolerance of repetition
Cookery:
Ability to follow written and verbal instructions
Accuracy
Speed of reaction
Ability to organise
Upper limb co-ordination
Strength and mobility
Responsibility
Initiative.

Activities in general
Oliver bicycle
Camden cycle
Treadle fret saw
Treadle sewing machine
Lathe
Metal work
Woodwork
Printing
Industrial work
Gardening
Clerical: writing and reading; typing; filing
Housecraft
Remedial games
Stool seating
Weaving: table loom; rug loom.

Length of treatment
This depends on the severity of the injury and the progression
of the patient in treatment.

Prognosis
Maximum recovery usually within 2 years.

Other treatment
Physiotherapy

Remedial gym
Speech therapy
Psychologist
Orthoptist.

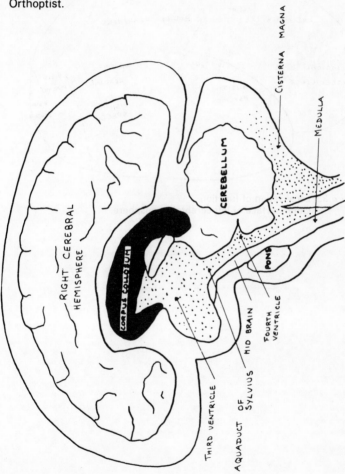

Figure 32 Diagram of sagital section through cerebral and cerebellar

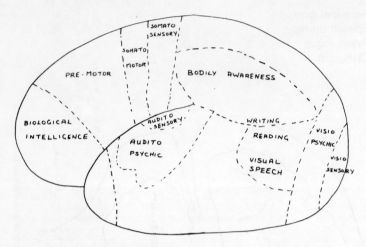

Figure 33 Localisation of function
Outer surface of left cerebral hemisphere

9 / PARKINSON'S SYNDROME

PARKINSON'S SYNDROME

It is degeneration of the globus pallidus, caudate nucleus, putamen and substantia nigra (see diagram).

Signs and symptoms
Rigidity
Inco-ordination
Festinating gait and difficulty initiating walking
Mask-like face
'Pin rolling' tremor, which continues while at rest, but stops on effort
Premature greying of the hair and ageing
Writing becomes small and illegible (micrographic)
Speech slow and monotonous owing to immobility of lips and tongue
Difficulty in swallowing, which leads to dribbling
Eyes: nystagmus and difficulty with accommodation
Mental changes: slowing of expressive ability; general slowing down leading to depression; blunting of mental ability.

Complication
Depression.

Precaution
Falling owing to instability.

Aims of treatment
1 Personal independence
2 Improve co-ordination

3 General mobility
4 Introduce a hobby or interest.

Functional assessment
Assessment:
   Pre-operative
   Post-operative
   Drug trials
Upper limb function test
Co-ordination
   (a) Follow through the maze with a pen
   (b) Place a dot in every square
Writing
Speech.

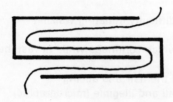

Figure 34

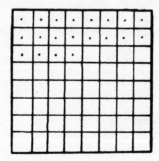

Figure 35

Aids to daily living

Suitable aids include:

 Loose clothing

 Front fastenings

 Non-slip shoe soles

 Aprons with weights in the pockets or bottom hem to
 prevent falling backwards or forwards

Allow plenty of time when eating

Check reactions, e.g. to the door bell ringing when cooking

Considerations after operation: wigs to aid appearance, and
 head scarves.

Home visit

Points to look for include:

 Slip mats should be checked

 Non-slip polish

 Rails beside the bath, lavatory, stairs, corridors

 Trolley with two wheels on the front and two stabilising legs
 at the back

 Labour saving devices.

Principles of treatment

1 Activities should be bilateral and relaxing

2 Large to fine activities to increase co-ordination

3 General mobility

4 Group work to boost morale.

Activities

Oliver bicycle to obtain a good walking pattern

Skittles for co-ordination and balance

Darts for socialisation and co-ordination of hand and eye

Gardening as a hobby

Weaving for large bilateral movements

Printing with the paper placed some distance away from the
 press

Composing in the late stages for co-ordination

Housework; cleaning

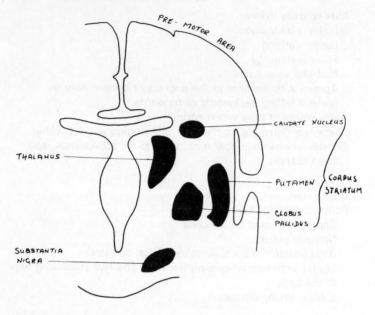

Figure 36 Transverse view

Cooking: to boost morale and to assess the patient's
   capabilities
Hand games: peggotty; draughts; solitaire; ball throwing
Sanding a large surface.

Prognosis
Parkinson's Syndrome is a degenerative condition therefore
   the prognosis will depend on the reaction to the treatment.

Other treatments
Drug trials
Surgery:
   Stereotactic (pallidectomy or pallidotomy) to reduce rigidity
   Thalamotomy to reduce tremor
Physiotherapy.

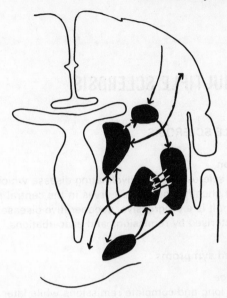

Figure 37 Chief connections of the corpus striatum

10 / MULTIPLE SCLEROSIS

MULTIPLE SCLEROSIS

Definition

Multiple sclerosis is a demyelinating disease which affects the myelin sheath around the nerves in the central nervous system. It is a progressive, degenerative disease and is characterised by remissions and exacerbations.

Signs and symptoms

Early stage
It shows long and complete remissions while later patients condition fluctuates to a small extent.

Early symptoms	Incidence
Weakness of control of limbs	50%
Visual symptoms: acute unilateral retrabulbar neuritis	29%
Sensory symptoms	11%
Miscellaneous, e.g. vertigo, tremor	10%

Other symptoms include
Dragging of one leg: paresis
Diplopia
Slurring of speech
Feeling of heaviness of the limbs.

Later as the disease progresses
Intention tremor
Ataxia
Incontinence/urgency

Inco-ordination
Dysarthria
Spasticity and contractions.

Mental symptoms may include
Euphoria
Emotional changes
Reduction in intellectual ability
Depression
Emotional lability
Delusions and terminal dementia are sometimes seen.

Prognosis

The course of the disease is extremely variable; it may
terminate fatally after 3 months, or the patient may be able
to work for 30 years after the onset
A relapse may last a life time, or the patient may recover
permanently from the first attack
The average duration of life in fatal cases is 20 years.

Treatment

There is no specific treatment. Fatigue is to be avoided, but
every effort should be made to keep the patient at his usual
occupation for as long as possible
Certain drugs will help: A.C.T.H., arsenic
Rest—exercise therapy. Physical exercise to patient's limit,
then complete rest
Surgery—spinal cord stimulation by electrical implant.

Aims of treatment

1 Maintain morale, particularly by emphasising what the
patient can do
2 Continual assessment of A.D.L.
3 Maintain and support the patient and his family
4 Maintain physical function.

First interview

Full first interview and assessment to give a sound picture of
each individual case:

(a) Check if the patient knows his diagnosis by reading the medical notes
(b) Discuss with the relatives, and recommend the Multiple Sclerosis Society
(c) Check job and home situation.

Early stage
A.D.L.
Cookery and light housework
Simple dressmaking, plus advice on adaptations to clothing
Typing
Basketry: to improve fine finger movement and co-ordination
Weaving
Pottery and clay modelling
Mosaics and large ceramics
Gardening
Archery
Painting
Work in groups to encourage socialisation:
    (a) industrial work
    (b) cards, e.g. bridge
    (c) scrabble and other table games.

Late stage
Aim: to build up morale and give support
1 Housework and cookery
2 Light carpentry
3 Establish mobility with sticks or a self-propelled wheelchair
4 Wheelchair assessment and practise
5 Job and job assessment
6 Home visit
7 The patient may need a P.O.S.S.U.M. in the later stages
8 Refer to the domiciliary occupational therapist who may give advice to the patient to attend a sheltered workshop.

Length of treatment
Intensive treatment until the patient is as independent as possible 6-8 week periods of treatment
Re-assessment after relapses.

Precautions and complications

1 Precaution against low morale by pushing the patient too hard
2 Check if the patient is aware of his diagnosis
3 Awareness of extensor spasm. Teach the patient how to relax
4 A restraining leg strap should be fitted to the wheelchair
5 Depending on the patients abilities, take care to choose activities carefully
6 Precaution regarding eyesight
7 Prevention of pressure sores.

Activities contra-indicated

1 Activities involving fine finger work in later stages
2 Carrying hot dishes
3 Activities should be carefully chosen considering symptoms presented, i.e. no cooking where a strong intention tremor is present.

The housewife with multiple sclerosis

Labour saving devices
Early independence training for the child
Educate other members of the family
Buy clothes which are easy to launder
Keep the child's hair a length which is easy to manage
Dress the child on the bed
Low bathroom stool for the child to stand on while being dressed
Old nursing chair for mother when handling the child
Shallow bath, or stool in the bath, or sink for bathing the child.

11 / OSTEO-ARTHROSIS

OSTEO-ARTHROSIS

(Osteo arthritis)

It is a chronic degenerative condition affecting the articular
 cartilage and adjacent bone. It may affect one, or many
 joints
It is commonly found in the hip and knee
It may also affect: spine; shoulder; elbows; thumb
It may occur at an early age as a result of trauma or abnormal
 strain, but generally occurs in the older person
Course of the condition:
 The cartilage is eroded and destroyed
 The bone is thickened
 There is narrowing of the joint space.

Signs and symptoms
Of the affected joint:
 Pain
 Stiffness
 Crepitus
 Deformity
 Restricted range
Nodules on the hands: Heberden's nodes.

Non-operative procedures
Drugs: mainly analgesics
Splintage: to prevent and correct deformity
Physiotherapy.

Operative procedures

Arthrodesis

Arthroplasty:

Hip: Austen Moore ⎫
       Thompson ⎬ head of femur replacement

       Charnley ⎫
       McKee Farrar ⎬ total hip replacement
       McKee Arden
       I.C.L.H. ⎭

Knee: Platt
       I.C.L.H.
       Waldius
       Shiers
       Freeman   hingeless

Osteotomy:

Hip: McMurray

Knee: Wedge
       Benjamin
       Brackett.

Complications

1 Limited hip flexion
2 Dislocation of the prosthesis
3 Shortening of the leg
4 May be a tendency for hip flexion contractures.

Precautions

1 There should be no adduction of the hip joint if a prosthesis
  has been inserted; check past-operative policy of surgeon
2 Do not over-mobilise the joint
3 Do not place additional strain on the other leg.

Aims of treatment

1 Increase the stability of the joint
2 Increase the mobility if possible
3 Personal independence
4 Diet should be controlled, i.e. the patient should not be
  over-weight.

Functional assessment

1 Measure joint range, particularly after an operation
2 Measure muscle bulk, particularly quadriceps
3 Sitting down in a chair and sitting tolerance
4 Standing up from a chair and standing tolerance
5 Ability to walk up and down steps
6 Walking, using an aid if necessary.

Aids to daily living

Labour saving devices and methods: e.g. Long handled
  dustpan.
  Time and motion study.
Chair should be raised for easy sitting and standing (or an
  ejector cushion used)
Dressing, e.g.:
  Use of stocking gutter
  Long handled shoe horn
  Long tapes on trousers and pants
  Front fastenings
  Elastic shoe laces
  Raglan sleeves
Bath, e.g.:
  Bath board
  Bath seat
  Non-slip mat
  Rails
Lavatory, e.g.:
  Raised seat
  Rails
Bed: should be raised to the level of the buttock crease if
  necessary
Stairs: rails on at least one side
Resting splints may be required to prevent deformity
Shoe raise may be required to correct leg shortening
Use of public transport if required
Getting in and out of a car.

Home visit

Points to look for should include

Paths: even surface
Steps: height
Ramps under the doors
Floor surfaces: non-slip
Mats: fixed
Height of switches: within reach
Type of heating: coal, central
Stairs: depth and rails
Bathroom: layout and heights.

Non-operative treatment
Aims
1 Increase stability of the joint
2 Increase mobility of the joints above and below the affected
  joint.

Early stage
A.D.L.
Treadle sewing machine
Treadle fretsaw
Weaving: using appropriate adaptations
Printing: using appropriate adaptations
Lathe
Oliver bicycle
Camden cycle
Remedial games:
   Football (seated)
   Foot noughts and crosses
   Skittles
   Shuffle board with the feet
   Outdoor draughts.

Middle stage
Housework, including labour saving methods
Gardening, e.g. digging and weeding
Treadle sewing machine
Treadle fretsaw with additional resistance
Printing with adaptations upgraded
Lathe upgraded by resistance and time

Oliver bicycle upgraded by resistance and time
Camden cycle upgraded by resistance and time
Remedial games:

Foot noughts and crosses

Skittles

Outdoor draughts.

Last stage
Work simulation.

Post-operative treatment

Early stage
A.D.L. (after arthroplasty: gradual withdrawal of aids and re-education of sitting and walking)
Weaving: using appropriate adaptations
Camden cycle
Treadle sewing machine
Treadle fretsaw
Fletcher-Wiltshire bed loom: for hip flexion and extension only
Remedial games:

Football (seated)

Shuffle board with the feet.

Middle stage
Camden cycle upgraded for range
Oliver bicycle
Lathe
Treadle sewing machine
Treadle fretsaw with resistance
Printing with suitable adaptations
Foot power loom
Housework
Remedial games:

Foot draughts

Skittles.

Late stage
Work simulation
Printing with adaptations upgraded

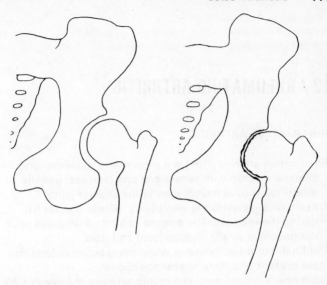

Figure 38 Osteo-arthrosis of the hip
(a) Normal bone structure of the hip
(b) Result of osteo-arthrosis of the hip
Points to note:
1 Eroded acetabulum
2 Eroded head of femur
3 Narrowing joint space
4 Adduction deformity

Housework: heavier activities
Gardening, e.g. digging and weeding
Tyre walking.

12 / RHEUMATOID ARTHRITIS

RHEUMATOID ARTHRITIS

Rheumatoid arthritis (R.A.) is a progressive inflammatory, bilateral disease with remissions and relapses, initially affecting synovial membranes in the smaller joints

Treatment is given during remissions as rest is essential during the relapses. The disease can attack all joints until the patient is totally incapacitated and rigid

The final 'burnt out' phase is when the residual deformities are present and there is absence of pain

Incidence: it occurs most commonly between the ages of 20 and 35 years and in women more than men. One in 50 of the population is affected and 5% are permanently disabled.

Signs and symptoms
Onset is usually insidious.

Early stage
Pain in joints
Hot and swollen joints
General malaise
Pyrexia
Anaemia
Loss of weight
Loss of energy.

Later stage
Stiffness especially in the morning
Restricted movement
Pain
Increasing deformities

Tenderness
Swelling
Weakness
Depression or euphoria.

Precautions

1 No treatment during relapses
2 Prevent contractures
3 Prevent further deformities
4 Avoid painful movement, and extreme of temperature
5 No static work
6 No gripping or twisting movements
7 Watch for hot and painful joints
8 When the patient is on steroid therapy, watch for oedema and sensitive skin condition.

Complications

1 There may be some paraesthesia
2 If the patient is receiving gold treatment there may be a rash.

Aims of treatment

1 Relief of pain
2 Personal independence
3 Maintain maximum level of function
4 Boost morale
5 Prevent deformity
6 Work assessment
7 Provide a hobby activity.

Functional assessment

A.D.L. and supply aids when necessary
Test the following:
　Observe the patient when taking off coat, hanging it up and doing up bottons
　Turning key in lock
　Cutting bread
　Walking and use of stairs
　Handling money: suggest use of tray purse

Picking up articles from the floor
Writing
Upper limb function test (see appendix)
Photographs can be taken of the deformity, especially if
    surgery is contemplated
Measure oedema, if present.

A.D.L.

Main points to be considered:
    Adapted handles
    Use of 'Velcro' on clothing
    Loose, light clothing
    Rails where necessary
    Sitting while washing and dressing
    Labour saving methods and equipment in the kitchen
    Home visit
    Wheelchair assessment.

Activities

Should be rhythmical and repetitive, allowing for rest periods.

Upper limb
Cooking: pastry, bread
Games: elevated; darts; quoits
Housework
Stool seating
Cord knotting
Paper sculpture
Gardening
Clay modelling
Printing unadapted.

Lower limb
Foot games
Upright rug loom weaving
Skittles
Oliver bicycle
Treadle fret-saw
Treadle sewing machine
Weaving: knee flexion and extension.

Deformities	Functional loss	Splint	Surgery
Swan neck	*Poor power Grip*		*Synovectomy EARLY Silastic hinges*
Ulnar drift	Weak grip Writing difficult Opposition weak Inability to lift Loss of M.P. extension as tendons are subluxed	M.U.D.	M.P. Joints arthrodesed in mid-flexion Tendons sutured onto extensor expansion
Boutonniere	Weakness of grip Difficulty with lifting	Resting splint	Suture of subluxed tendons
Egg cup erosion	Stiff fingers		Prosthetic M.C. heads
Subluxation	Weak hand Instability of joint		Silastic hinges
Hyper-extension of thumb	No pinch grip		I.P. joint arthrodesed in partial flexion
Subluxed wrist	Grip and movement limited	Resting splint	Arthrodesis in functional position
Subluxed M.T.P. joints	Flat feet Poor walking pattern	Insole built up at instep	
Spindle shaped joints	Limited and weak flexion		
Singleton- one extensor tendon out of alignment	Loss of extension of the one affected finger		Tendon is sutured into extensor expansion

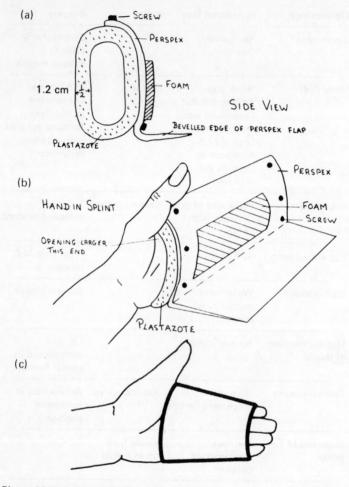

(a)
SCREW
PERSPEX
FOAM
1.2 cm ½"
SIDE VIEW
BEVELLED EDGE OF PERSPEX FLAP
PLASTAZOTE

(b)
HAND IN SPLINT
PERSPEX
FOAM
SCREW
OPENING LARGER THIS END
PLASTAZOTE

(c)

Figure 39 Splints for lifting plates
One used on each hand to aid in lifting plates
by resting crockery on perspex flap
(a) Side view
(b) Hand in splint
(c) Shape of hand piece

13 / AMPUTEES

AMPUTEES

Types

1 Traumatic: when the damage following an accident is irrepairable
2 Congenital: in certain malformations, where normal function cannot be obtained
3 Nerve lesions: when sensation has not returned after a period of two years and the limb is not likely to be functional
4 Infection: such as osteo-myelitis, which had produced a deformity
5 Peripheral vascular deficiency: as occurs commonly with diabetes, is the most common indication for amputation because of pain due to ischaemia or gangrene.

Complications

1 Hip contracture: flexion and either adduction or abduction according to the level of amputation
2 Knee flexion contracture
3 Skin breakdown.

Precautions

1 Hypersensitivity
2 Rubbing of harness on the body
3 Excessive sweating due to diminished body surface area.

Diabetic amputations (Peripheral vascular deficiency)
Precautions
1 Diet: this should be enforced

117

2 Do not over-work the other limb

3 Contra-indicate the use of tight corsets because of venous insufficiency

4 Take particular care of skin on the stump and on the other limb

5 Prevent rubbing of the stump: advise the patient to use two stump socks

6 Temporary prostheses and other prosthesis should be ischial bearing.

Aims of treatment

Boost morale

Toughening of stump, e.g. by percussion

Personal independence

Increase mobility

Strengthen residual part of limb and other limb

Correct use and care of prosthesis

Prevent contractures

Increase tolerance to prosthesis

Work assessment.

First interview

Morale: give realistic information to boost morale and to eliminate undue fears, e.g. fears about marriage and employment

Examine stump and explain about care of the skin, and show the patient how to bandage the stump (see diagrams)

Explain about phantom sensations: sensation of pain or itching in amputated limb

Check range of movement

Check sensation and hypersensitivity

Check financial situation, job and compensation

Arrange a home visit and wheelchair assessment if necessary.

Stump bandaging

The stump is bandaged to prevent oedema and maintain good stump shape after operation therefore it makes fitting for the prosthesis easier; also the skin is not flabby and will not rub and become sore

The bandage is elasticated; it must be applied with even
   tension but *not* tightly; pressure being concentrated on the
   sides of the stump end to push fluid upwards. Pressure
   should not be concentrated on the end of the stump itself,
   nor constrict more proximally as this will encourage oedema
The patient should be taught to reapply the bandage as it
   loosens.

Method

1 Begin bandaging on the anterior aspect of the stump. Bring
   the bandage straight down the middle, asking the patient to
   hold the top of the bandage with both hands

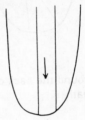

Figure 40 Anterior aspect

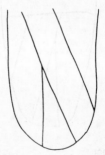

Figure 41 Posterior aspect

2 Take the bandage up the posterior aspect of the stump
   Fold the bandage back on itself and bring it down the leg
   again, diagonally
   Ask the patient to hold this

3 Bring the bandage tightly round the lower end of the stump,
and pass it diagonally across the anterior aspect of the
stump

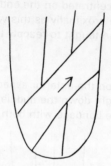

Figure 42 Anterior aspect

4 Wind the bandage around the back of the stump, securing
the first fold underneath

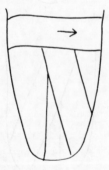

Figure 43 Posterior aspect

5 Wind the bandage diagonally across the front, concentrating
the pressure on the lower edge
The arrows show the areas to which it is most important to
apply pressure

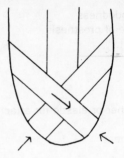

Figure 441 Anterior aspect

6 Wind the bandage around the stump once to secure the
ends
Then continue a figure of eight
The more the bandage is overlapped, the tighter it lies at
the corners and therefore is more effective
It can be wound round horizontally at intervals, but too
many of these will lead to a bulbous stump.

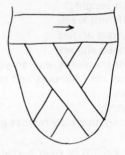

Figure 45 Posterior aspect

UPPER LIMB AMPUTEES

Aims of treatment
Prevent a frozen shoulder

Prevent 'one handedness'
Teach correct use of prosthesis
Work assessment.

Pre-prosthetic

Check A.D.L.

Provide cuff: leather or elastic for attachment of tools and appliances:

Writing equipment

Eating utensils

Table tennis bat

Tools, e.g. plane

Paint brush

Kitchen utensils.

Post-prosthetic

Check use of prosthesis, how to put it on and how to use the terminal device

Practise specific things:

Use of different weights

Working at different levels

Working at various angles

Picking up various shapes

Use of different pressures, e.g. an egg or a golf ball

Use of switches, door handles and taps

Writing practice

A.D.L. instruction:

Avoid tight clothing; this may restrict good function of the prosthesis

Recommend the patient to wear a vest under the harness to prevent any rubbing

Dress by putting clothing onto the prosthesis first

For the above elbow amputee with a prosthesis, it may be easier to have the elbow joint flexed when dressing to prevent the garment from slipping. Alternatively have the elbow locked in extension, pull up clothes to shoulder and hold under arm.

Activities
Car cleaning
Cookery for various grips/angles/weights
General bi-lateral activities of daily living
Kitchen activities
Ironing
Housework
Elevated draughts
Fine solitaire for fine grip and release
Functional activities:
  Use of keys
  Opening doors
  Picking up matches
  Pouring out water
  Picking up money
  Winding a watch
  Turning a tap
  Doing up shoe laces
  Opening a safety pin
Window-box gardening: use of various grades and weights of
  tools
Jig-saws with large pieces
Meccano for fine work with nuts and bolts
Leather work
Balsa wood work
Planing and sawing
Sanding
Table Tennis
Weaving: rug loom
Window cleaning.

LOWER LIMB AMPUTEE

Aims of treatment
Encourage a good walking pattern
Standing/sitting tolerance
Encourage balance
Personal independence.

Pre-prosthetic—above knee amputation
Activities with a temporary prosthesis or
temporary wheelchair
A.D.L.

Teach correct walking pattern with crutches
Stair practice using upstairs facilities
Transfers

Other activities:

Lathe: to build up quadriceps muscles. Initially sitting on a
Camden stool and later standing
Bench work: for standing tolerance and balance
Cross-cut sawing: for standing tolerance and balance
Dancing: for balance and socialisation
Gardening: for balance, standing tolerance, bending and
walking over rough ground
Treadle fret-saw
Treadle sewing machine
Archery
Darts
Table tennis   For balance, standing tolerance,
Bowls   stooping, bending and socialisation
Snooker
Foot O's and X's.

Without temporary prosthesis or pylon
Table games: patient lying prone to prevent flexion
contractures of the hip
Fletcher-Wiltshire bed loom: for all hip movements
Printing: with hip extension adaptation
Upper limb activities for strengthening
Activities while seated on a Camden stool:

Benchwork
Metal work
Stool seating
Printing unadapted
Teach stump bandaging
Dressing
Lavatory: rails may be needed.

Post-prosthetic

Check stump

Check use of prosthesis, how to put it on, and general
care

A.D.L. instruction: avoid tight clothing.

Activities

As for the temporary prosthesis, encouraging a good walking
pattern

Work assessment.

Below knee amputee

Pre-prosthetic—no pylon yet supplied

A.D.L.

Transfers

Dressing

Lavatory

Bathing

Percussion of stump

Vibration activities

Reciprocal quads on lathe and at the bench

Weaving and printing with extension lag adaptations.

Post-prosthetic—also post-pylon

A.D.L.:

Dressing

Transfers

Putting on prosthesis and its care

Walking practice e.g. archery

Practice on stairs and public transport.

Other activities

Lathe work: standing

Oliver bicycle

Darts and quoits for standing tolerance and balance

Benchwork: standing

Weaving: knee flexion/extension adaptation

Printing: knee flexion/extension adaptation

Walking practice: including walking on uneven ground

Digging: for balance and standing tolerance
Archery
Cross-cut sawing
Foot games.

Clothing for lower limb amputees

Loose fitting, hard wearing fabric
Waist bands sometimes need to be a size larger to fit over the
harness of the prosthesis.

Dressing method

1 Put on vest
2 Put trousers and underpants on prosthesis
3 Put prosthesis on with foot of prosthesis externally rotated,
  fasten harness and foot will turn to central position
4 Put other leg through underpants and trousers
5 Pull up and fasten at waist
6 Continue dressing in normal way.

Clothing for the amputee

Points to look for when choosing clothes for a bilateral
amputee, to encourage greater independence:

1 General:
  All clothes should be loose fitting; avoid tight armholes
  Reinforce any place where there is friction against part of
  the prosthesis
  Look for easy fastenings (zips, Velcro, large trouser hooks)
  Look for extra fullness to allow for strain when operating a
  split hook
2 Coats:
  Loose fitting without a belt
  Wide sleeves, deep armholes
  Buttons: flat, sewn on with a thread shank
3 Shirts:
  Jacket styles with front fastenings
  Avoid styles that do up too high at the neck
  Replace small buttons with larger ones
  Sports shirts outside trousers avoid the difficulty of tucking in

4 Trousers:
Zip in fly, with split ring on tab
Large trouser hook or Velcro at waist, or elastic insets at waist with no fastenings
5 Sweaters:
Cardigans are much easier to manage than sweaters.

14 / BURNS

BURNS

Wallace's rule of 9

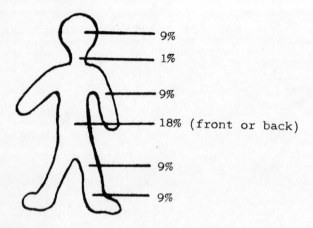

9%

1%

9%

18% (front or back)

9%

9%

Figure 46

Burns may be superficial or deep; 1st, 2nd or 3rd degree.

Types
1 Chemicals, e.g. acid and alkaline
2 Scalds
3 Extreme heat or cold
4 Radiation
5 Friction.

Signs and symptoms
Shock
Fluid loss
Tissue loss
Sensation loss
Pain.

Complications
1 Infection
2 Contractures
3 Adhesions
4 Scarring
5 Donor area
6 Personality change and low morale.

Precautions
1 Friction: therefore pad tools, or wear a cotton glove
2 Excessive perspiration
3 De-sensitisation
4 Initially avoid heat and damp.

Aims of treatment
1 Reduce oedema
2 Prevent contractures, by the use of splints if necessary or elastic garments (Jobst garments)
3 Maintain morale, by the use of cosmetics and group activities
4 Maintain or increase movements
5 Toughen skin
6 Sensation training
7 Personal independence and work assessment.

Functional assessment
This will depend on the burnt area
1 Check movement and measure
2 Check sensation
3 Find out attitude to burn and work

4 Is there a pending compensation claim?
5 A.D.L. check, especially if hands are involved.
(Home visit will depend on the individual.)

Principles of treatment

1 Bilateral
2 Wide
3 Elevated
4 Reverberating
5 Toughening
6 Tolerance to heat and friction
7 Stereognosis and sensation re-training
8 If there are contractures, exercise against the contracture
9 Groups for morale and discussion
10 Recreation
11 Work assessment
12 Application of orthoplast splintage
13 Application of body stockings.

Activities

Upper limb, early stage
Ball and hand games
Cards
Cat's cradle and other string games
Cord knotting: nitrim
Guillotining
Origami
Painting
Peggoty
Printing: unadapted
Sensation, e.g. dominoes
Skittles
Solitaire, e.g. marbles
Stereognosis training—identifying objects by touch
Table tennis
Typing
Wire twister
Writing.

Upper limb, later stage
Archery
Bilateral sander
Carpentry
Clay modelling
Cooking
Cord knotting: macrame
Industrial work
Paper sculpture
Printing: bell rope
Stool seating elevated: seagrass
Upright rug loom
Wire twister.

Lower limb
Ankle rotator
Bench work
Cross cut sawing
Gardening
Lathe
Noughts and crosses
Oliver bicycle
Printing: adapted
Table tennis
Treadle fretsaw
Treadle sewing machine
Tyre walking
Weaving: adapted
Wobble board.

Length of treatment
Daily of increasing duration
If no graft, treat for three weeks
If graft, treat for one month after each operation.

Other treatment
Nursing care:
  Plasma drip
  Dressings

Sterile air
Physiotherapy
Remedial gym
Surgery:
1 Grafts: needed when a skin defect is too large to be closed by direct suture
   (a) Full thickness graft: flap graft; free skin graft
   (b) Split skin graft
2 Z plasty: used to break the tension of a long scar and to release contractures.

15 / JOINT EXAMINATION

JOINT EXAMINATION

(a) Look at the joint
(b) Observe:
Skin:
    Bruising
    Drying, flaking (after plaster)
    Colour: cyanosis or inflammation
    Scarring
    Temperature
Oedema
Muscle wasting:
    The patient stands against the light so that outline of the
    body shows unilateral wasting
    (c) Joint measurement
This can either be exact or functional.

Functional activities for testing joint range

Ankle
Plantar and dorsiflexion:
    Standing on tip toe
    Crouching
    Walking: on rough ground; up stairs
    Ladder
    Standing in in/eversion.

Knee
Way the patient walks into the department
Going up a step (on and off a bus)
Stairs

Bending down to pick up an object
Doing up shoe laces
Climbing a ladder.

Hip
Sitting and standing
Stairs
Sitting tying shoe laces
Getting into a bath
Standing on one leg: abductors.

Hand
Undoing screw top jar
Turning a tap
Buttons
Undoing a safety pin
Strike a match
Turn a key in lock
Handling money
Pouring water
Turning over a page
Writing
Dialling telephone
Tying shoe laces
Handling knife, fork and spoon
Threading a needle
Rolling pastry
Picking up various sized objects, e.g. egg, ball etc.

Elbow
Flexion:
  Combing hair
  Drinking
  Shaving
Extension:
  Putting on shoe
  Picking up object when sitting down
  Reaching up to a shelf.

Pronation of forearm
Turning a door knob

Using a screw driver
Turning tap on and off
Turning key in lock.

Shoulder
Internal rotation:
  Tucking in shirt
  Tie on apron
  Doing up bra
  Doing up back zip
External rotation:
  Brushing hair
  Hook on back of dress
  Turning down collar
  Doing up back zip
Extension:
  Putting on coat
  Doing up zip
Flexion:
  Hanging up washing
  Hanging up coat
  Turning on light switch
  Putting things on shelf.

NAME	

HIP (tick unaffected range in colour code)

RIGHT RANGE		✓	LEFT RANGE		
Extension	Flexion		Flexion		Extension

Abduction	Adduction	Adduction	Abduction

	R. Leg under L. Leg	L. Leg under R. Leg	

DATE	Colour coded	29.4.1973

NAME	

KNEE (tick unaffected range in colour code)

RIGHT RANGE	✓	LEFT RANGE	
Flexion	Extension	Extension	Flexion

QUADRICEPS above knee 2" 5cm 4" 10cm	Above Patella	Patella	Below Patella	Calf	QUADRICEPS above knee 2" 5cm 4" 10cm	Above Patella	Patella	Below Patella	Calf
16" 42cm 19" 48cm	15" 37cm	14" 35cm	13" 33cm	14" 35cm	15" 37cm 17½" 45cm	15½" 40cm	15" 37cm	14" 35cm	13" 33cm

DATE	colour coded	30·4·73		

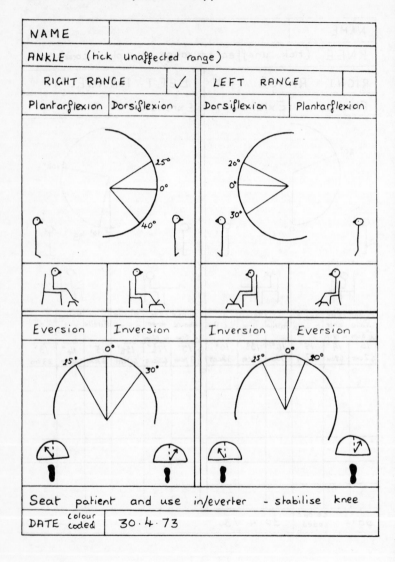

NAME							
DATE colour coded	30·4·73						
FOOT SWELLING (tick unaffected range)							
RIGHT RANGE			✓	LEFT RANGE			
1" 2.5cm above malleoli	Malleoli	Forefoot	H.T. heads	1" 2.5cm above malleoli	Malleoli	Forefoot	H.T. heads
8½" 22 cm	9" 23 cm	9" 23 cm	8½" 22 cm	9½" 24 cm	9½" 24 cm	9½" 24 cm	9" 23 cm

SHOULDER (tick unaffected range)	NAME				
LEFT RANGE		RIGHT RANGE			✓

Measure Bilaterally

Flexion	Extension	Abduction	Abduction	Extension	Flexion

DATE Colour Coded	Internal Rotation	External Rotation	External Rotation	Internal Rotation	NOTES
30. 4. 1973					Swelling Muscle Wasting
					Swelling - None
					Deltoid wasted

Arm Supported and horizontal

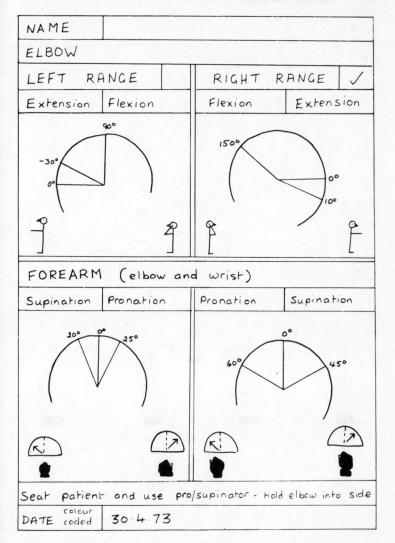

NAME	

ELBOW

LEFT RANGE			RIGHT RANGE	✓
Extension	Flexion		Flexion	Extension

FOREARM (elbow and wrist)

Supination	Pronation	Pronation	Supination

Seat patient and use pro/supinator - hold elbow into side

DATE	colour coded	30·4·73

NAME	

WRIST (tick unaffected range)

LEFT RANGE		RIGHT RANGE	✓
Extension	Flexion	Flexion	Extension

Left: 20°, 0°, 30°

Right: 70°, 0°, 80°

Rest patients forearm along the back of a chair or table

Ulnar Deviation	Radial Deviation	Radial Deviation	Ulnar Deviation

Left: 5° 0° 10°

Right: 30° 0° 30°

Rest patients hand and forearm on a table

SPAN (tip of thumb to tip of little finger)

6″ 15cm	8″ 20cm

Date	Colour coded	1 5. 73

NAME					
DYNAMOMETER RECORD (Tick unaffected hand)					
INDICATE SIZE OF BULB USED	LEFT HAND		RIGHT HAND	✓	
	DATE	POWER GRIP	PINCER GRIP	POWER GRIP	PINCER GRIP
M	1.5.73	2 lb 0.900 Kg		10 lb 4.5 Kg	

NAME	
THUMB (tick unaffected)	

LEFT RANGE		RIGHT RANGE	✓
Abduction		Abduction	

Extension		Extension	

Opposition		Opposition	
Distance from	2" 5cm	Distance from	0" 0cm
tip of thumb		tip of thumb	
to base of little finger		to base of little finger	
DATE colour coded	1.5.73		

NAME	

THUMB (continued) (tick unaffected range)

LEFT. RANGE		RIGHT RANGE	✓
Flexion		Flexion	
Carpometacarpal Joint		Carpometacarpal Joint	

0°
5°

0°
15°

| Metacarpophalangeal Joint | | Metacarpophalangeal Joint | |

0°
13°

0°
50°

| Interphalangeal Joint | | Interphalangeal Joint | |

0°
70°

0°
80°

DATE Colour Coded	1.5.1973

NAME									
FINGERS (tick unaffected)									
LEFT RANGE					RIGHT RANGE				✓
Finger spread	H.C.P. Flexion				H.C.P. Flexion				Finger spread
Distance from tips									Distance from tips
of indicated fingers									of indicated fingers
Little to mid = 4" 10cm									Little to mid = 6" 15cm
	Index	Mid	Ring	Little	Index	Mid	Ring	Little	
	80°	80°	80°	90°	90°	90°	90°	90°	
DATE Colour coded	2. 5. 73.								

NAME																
FINGERS (tick unaffected)																
LEFT RANGE								RIGHT RANGE								✓
Distal Interphalangeal Joint				Proximal Interphalangeal Jt				Proximal Interphalangeal J				Distal Interphalangeal Joint			

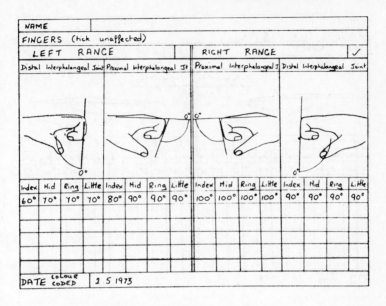

Index	Mid	Ring	Little	Index	Mid	Ring	Little	Index	Mid	Ring	Little	Index	Mid	Ring	Little
60°	70°	70°	70°	80°	90°	90°	90°	100°	100°	100°	100°	90°	90°	90°	90°
DATE COLOUR CODED		2 5 1973													

NAME																							

FINGERS (tick unaffected)

LEFT RANGE | RIGHT RANGE ✓

Extension | Extension

M.C.P extension >45° / DIP + PIP hyperextension only

M.C.P extension >45° / DIP + PIP hyperextension only

M.C.P				P.I.P				D.I.P				D.I.P				P.I.P				M.C.P			
Index	Mid	Ring	Little	Index	Mid	Ring	Little	Index	Mid	Ring	Little	Index	Mid	Ring	Little	Index	Mid	Ring	Little	Index	Mid	Ring	Little
10°	10°	-10°	-30°	0°	0°	-45°	-50°	0°	0°	-50°	-60°	8°	10°	10°	8°	0°	0°	0°	0°	45°	45°	40°	35°
				✓	✓																		

DATE Colour coded | 2.5.1973

APPENDIX
WEAVING ADAPTATIONS

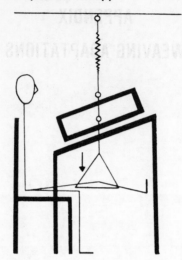

Figure 47 Extension lag

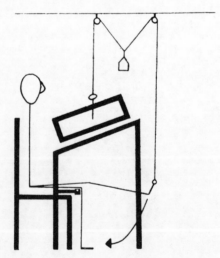

Figure 48 Knee flexion

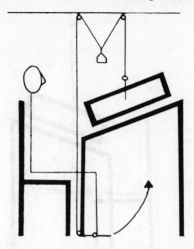

Figure 49 Knee extension

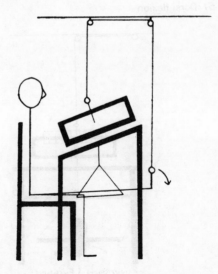

Figure 50 Plantar flexion

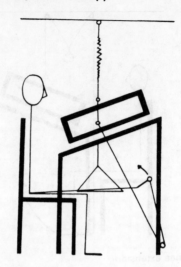

Figure 51 Dorsi flexion

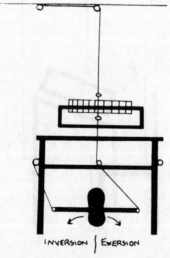

INVERSION | EVERSION

Figure 52 Adaptation shown for left leg

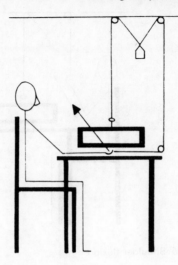

Figure 53 Elbow flexion

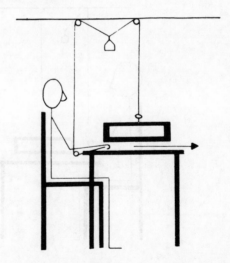

Figure 54 Elbow extension

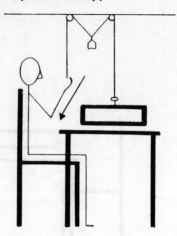

Figure 55 Shoulder flexion

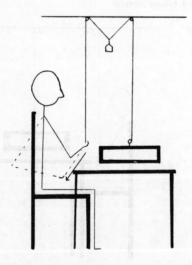

Figure 56 Shoulder extension

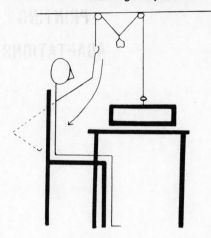

Figure 57 Shoulder flexion and extension

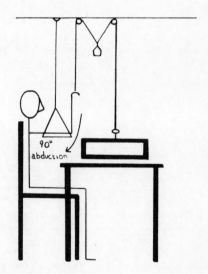

Figure 58 Shoulder rotation

PRINTING
ADAPTATIONS

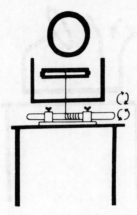

Figure 59 F.E.P.S.
   Wrist: flexion; extension
   Cylinder grip

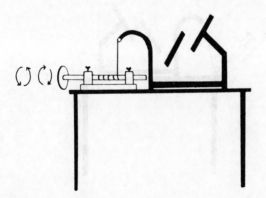

Figure 60 Disc: pronation and supination; span; I.P. flexion

Figure 61 Finger extension board

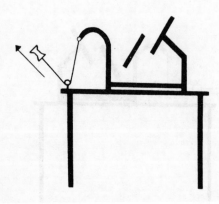

Figure 62 Cotton reel adaptation: isolation of little and ring finger
flexion

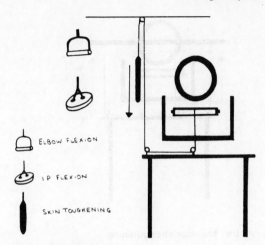

ELBOW FLEXION

I P FLEXION

SKIN TOUGHENING

Figure 63 Grips in elevation

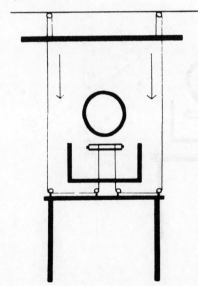

Figure 64 Double overhead bar: shoulder flexion; elbow flexion and extension

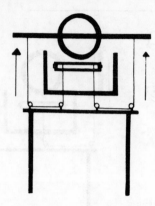

Figure 65 Double bar: shoulder strengthening

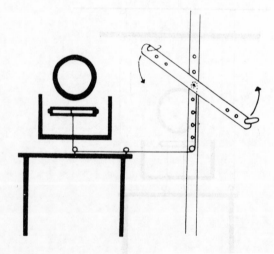

Figure 66 S.H.E.A.F.E.
abduction; flexion; extension
Elbow: flexion; extension

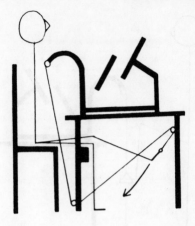

Figure 67 Knee flexion

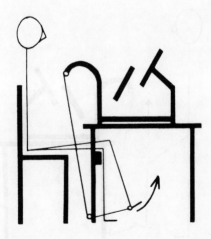

Figure 68 Knee extension

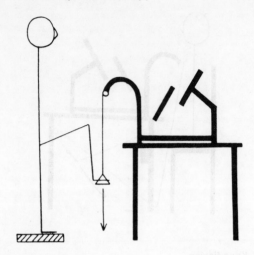

Figure 69 Knee extension

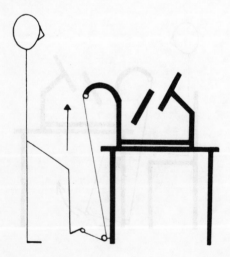

Figure 70 Hip and knee flexion

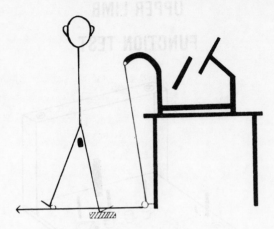

Figure 71 Hip abduction

UPPER LIMB

FUNCTION TEST

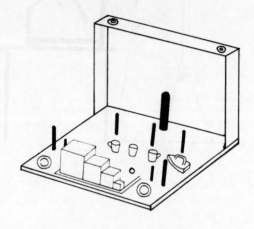

Fig 72 Upper limb function test (pipes and balls omitted from diagram)

UPPER LIMB FUNCTION TEST

Name	Date		Hand dominance	

Basic function	Right	Left

Grasp
  1 block 4" (10 cm)
  2 block 3" (7.5 cm)
  3 block 2" (5 cm)
  4 block 1" (2.5 cm)

Grip
  5 pipe 1¾" (4.5 cm)
  6 pipe ¾" (1.8 cm)

Pinch
  7 ball 3" (7.5 cm)

Marble 1" (2.5 cm)
  8 Index finger and thumb
  9 Middle ring finger and thumb
10 Ring finger and thumb
11 Small finger and thumb.

Ball bearing—½" (1.2 cm)
12 Index finger and thumb
13 Middle finger and thumb
14 Ring finger and thumb
15 Little finger and thumb.

Ball bearing—¼" (0.6 cm)
16 Index finger and thumb
17 Middle finger and thumb
18 Ring finger and thumb
19 Little finger and thumb.

Basic function	Right	Left

Placing
20 Washer over nail
21 Iron to shelf.

Supination and pronation
22 Pour water from pitcher to glass
23 Pour water from glass to glass (pro.)
24 Pour water back to first glass (sup.).

---

25 Place hand behind head
26 Place hand behind back
27 Hand to mouth.

Does pain interfere with function?
Is performance impeded by vision?

	81	81

Scoring
3 — performs test normally
2 — completes test, but takes abnormally long time or has great difficulty
1 — performs test partially
0 — can perform no part of test at all.

UPPER LIMB FUNCTION TEST

1 The patient is seated at the table with the shoulders at the same height as the shelf
2 Upper limbs are tested one at a time
3 For right upper limb:
  Have all objects on right side of board. See accompanying sheet:

1–4 place on shelf
5–6 place over uprights in the centre of the board
7 place in tray on right hand side of shelf
8–19 place in tray on right hand side of shelf
20–21 as described
22–27 as described
4 For left upper limb:
Repeat test with objects on the left hand side.

Object of test

All patients who are referred to the Occupational Therapy
Department with upper limb disabilities should be tested.
This assessment of their condition can later be used as a
comparison when the test is repeated for clinic attendance,
on discharge, or when resettlement is considered.

N.B. This test does not show how much the patient *is* using
the arm; this point is relevant in cases of sensory loss and
ignoral.

To test:
Strength
Mobility
Hand/eye co-ordination
Grip
Finger dexterity.

HOME VISIT
CHECK LIST

THE HOME VISIT

When making an initial home visit the following points should be taken into consideration

1 Type of dwelling
(a) House
(b) Flat: basement; ground floor; first floor
(c) Bungalow
(d) Lodgings
(e) Warden unit
(f) Who owns the property; will they allow adaptations

2 Patient lives
(a) Alone
(b) With spouse
(c) With children
(d) With other relatives
(e) With friends

3 Vicinity of home
(a) Countryside
(b) Village
(c) Town
(d) Distance to shops; P.O. etc.

4 Access to dwelling
(a) Garden gate: can patient manage this
(b) Path to entrance: good; dangerous surface; wide enough for wheelchair; steps; slopes; handrails needed
(c) Entrance: steps; handle; key

5 Mobility within the home
(a) Narrow passages: negotiable with walking frame or wheelchair
(b) Width of doorways
(c) Stairs: too steep; too narrow; handrails
(d) Access to kitchen; old houses usually have steps down to kitchen: hand grip; ramp

(e) Lighting: poor lighting is a potential hazard to the elderly and the partially sighted
(f) Floor covering: loose mats; worn carpets; slippery surfaces
(g) Seating: too high; too low; blocks; geriatric type chair
(h) Type of space heating e.g. paraffin; bottled gas; electric.

Specific rooms

1 *Hall*
Is there a telephone; can the patient use it

2 *Sitting room*
(a) Fire: type, can patient control knobs, light fire, get coal
(b) Light switches; sockets

3 *Kitchen*
(a) General layout: is space used economically; switches; meters
(b) Work heights, cooker height, sink height
(c) Cupboard heights
(d) Trolley
(e) Hatchway to dining room
(f) Windows: how do they open
(g) Taps
(h) Assess ability to cope with meal preparation: most of this can be done verbally.

4 *Bathroom*
(a) Up or down stairs
(b) Is lavatory accessible
(c) Seat height
(d) Independence aids: handgrips; vertical rails; horizontal rails; raised seat
(e) Bath: can patient get in and out; bath seat; bath board; bath mat; rails; hoist
(f) Shower unit installed thermostatically controlled
(g) Taps: can patient manage them

5 *Bedroom*
(a) Assess patient's ability to get in and out of bed; height

(b) Independence aids: monkey bar; rails; rope ladder; blocks; hoist
(c) Fracture board: if too soft
(d) Commode
(e) Bedding.

DOMICILIARY ASSESSMENT

Aim
To assess the problems facing a patient after discharge from hospital

Pre-visit preparation
Assessment of the patient should commence before seeing him at home
Obtain as much information as possible about the patient prior to home visit.

Sources of information
1 Consultant and medical staff
2 Ward sister
3 Physiotherapist
4 Social worker
5 G.P.
6 Health Clinic; health visitor; community nurse
7 Patient's friends and relatives
8 The patient himself
9 Social Services Department.

Arrangements
The occupational therapist should make prior arrangement for a relative or friend of the patient to unlock the door on the day of the visit.

Disabilities and chief reasons for domiciliary visit
1 Hemiplegics:
   Kitchen organisation

Toilet management
Ability to get in and out of bed, bath and chair
Stairs

2 Paraplegic:
Wheelchair management in the house
Transfers: bath; toilet; chair; bed
Labour saving techniques in the kitchen

3 Quadraplegic:
Instruct relatives on lifting techniques
Management of hoists

4 Elderly Frail
Kitchen management
Toilet management
Bed, bath, chair
Stairs

5 Multiple sclerosis:
Parkinson's syndrome:
Safety devices
Work organisation
Stairs

6 Rheumatoid arthritis:
Osteoarthrosis:
Mobility
Stairs if lower limb affected
Toilet; bath; bed; chair
Kitchen management.

Community services

1 Home help; how often; what duties does she do
2 Community nurse; for bathing; medical care: dressings; injections
3 Health Clinic: health visitor
4 Chiropodist
5 Over 60's club
6 Meals on wheels
7 Voluntary services
8 Social Services Department
9 Department of Health and Social Security allowances

Special equipment

1 Aids to mobility: walking stick; tripod; quadrapod; walking frame; wheelchair
2 Hoists: mobile or electric
3 Allowances for mobility
4 Housebound equipment: radio, T.V. telephone

Referrals for home help, community nurse, health visitors, meals on wheels, should be sent to the social worker.

WHEEL CHAIR
CHECK LIST

WHEELCHAIRS

Types of patient who may require a wheelchair

1 The elderly, through general arthritis
   The chair may be required for both indoor and outdoor use
   especially when senior citizen holidays are arranged
2 R.A.: according to the extent of disability from the disease
   May require an outdoor or indoor chair or both
3 Cerebral palsy children: often require special chairs and
   usually need numerous adaptations, e.g. back extensions,
   strappings, ball bearing support
4 Severe cardiac and respiratory diseases where exercise is
   limited
5 Degenerative diseases: M.S., Parkinsonism, muscular
   dystrophy
   Possible only outdoor chair required at first, progressing to
   an indoor
6 Amputees: lower limb amputees often have the large wheel
   at the front, but this is not good for posture and not
   recommended; or have rear wheels set back 3″ for stability
   All bi-lateral lower limb amputees supplied with a
   wheelchair
7 Hemiplegics: those unable to walk far require an outdoor
   chair, they may require a one arm drive wheelchair for
   indoor use
8 Paraplegics.

Assessment for wheelchairs
Name   Address
Age
Weight
Height

Does patient already have a wheelchair
If so, is it privately owned, hired or loaned
If on loan, from whom.

Is wheelchair required for indoor use
Does patient have any steps indoors

Where are these steps
What is the width of the narrowest doorway
What is the width of the passage outside this doorway
What is the width of the narrowest part of the passage that
   the chair must go through
How does patient get indoors.

Is wheelchair required for outdoor use
If so, are there steps at the front or back door
Can patient manage to get up and down these steps
Does patient live on street level
If not, is there a lift
If no lift, can patient get up and down the stairs
How many flights of stairs must patient climb
Has the patient somewhere to keep the chair on street level
Could someone take the chair up or downstairs
Who could help with the chair
What is the width of the narrowest passage through which
   the chair must pass
Is the district in which the patient lives hilly
Is the wheelchair to go into a car
If so, which model is the car
Does patient go to a club or day centre regularly, if so, do they
   have transport.

ASSESSING FOR A WHEELCHAIR

Each year about 70,000 wheelchairs are issued by the
Department of Health and Social Security and currently
nearly 230,000 wheelchairs are being used in England
alone. A very high proportion issued are not the most
suitable available for the patient.

Classification of wheelchairs
1 Folding or rigid
2 Self propelled, pushed or car transit chairs
3 Indoor or outdoor chairs
4 Standard weight or light weight chairs

5 Outsize, adult, junior or child size.

Folding self propelled chairs are the standard general purpose chairs (model 8 range). Indoor chairs are designed for easy manoeuvreability and include toilet chairs. Outdoor chairs are designed to be pushed by an attendant and consequently have comfortable upholstery, sprung frame, retractable foot board, detachable arms and an apron

Car transit chairs are easily folded, but are not suitable for pushing long distances or over soft or rough ground

Standard weight chairs (50 lbs 22.23 kg upwards) are robust and necessary for continuous or heavy use. Light weight chairs (36 lbs 16.32 Kg) are suitable for patients under 16 stone (101.60 Kg) or for occasional use only

Front wheel self propelled wheelchairs are the most easily managed for indoor use on carpets, but the wheels impede side transfers and close forward approach

Rear wheel self propelled chairs can negotiate curbs and are more suitable for outdoor and general use, front wheel chairs cannot be tilted by an attendant.

Features

Frames

Single cross-brace chairs will allow a direct approach up to and partially over a toilet. Most ministry chairs have a double cross-brace.

Wheels

Most general purpose ministry chairs have 22" (559 mm) pneumatic rear wheels, but sizes of wheels need to be varied according to space available at home and the patients special needs. If specified, rear wheels can be 20", 22", or 24" (508 mm, 559 mm or 610 mm) in diameter. Bigger wheels are easier to reach and turn, but may present problems for sideways transfer

Tyres may be solid or pneumatic. Solid tyres are easier to negotiate indoors over carpets; pneumatic tyres are easier out of doors, do not slip on wet surfaces and give more comfort

Castor wheels are usually 7" (178 mm) in diameter and solid, but they can be varied, i.e. spokes for lightness (less robust) or pneumatic for out of doors

Hand rims with capstans may be fitted to any size wheels for patients who cannot grip the standard rim, but they are difficult to manoeuvre in restricted spaces.

Backrests

On all ministry chairs the backrests are tilted between 5 and 25 degrees from vertical. The most common 15 degrees. Too great an angle can make a patient slide forward in the seat and be a cause of inability to propel the chair. Backrest extensions are available in various heights

On light weight chairs, folding backrests are available, this aids folding and loading in confined spaces.

Footrests

1 Fixed
2 Retractable
3 Divided for easy access to chair
4 Swinging detachable: for removal for use in a confined space
5 Bolt on elevating leg rests
6 Swinging detachable elevating leg rests
7 Heel loops, check straps and heel restraining fitments.

All footrests on folding chairs are adjustable with a spanner.

Arms

1 Fixed
2 Detachable: for sideways transfers
3 Domestic arms: for close forward approach
4 Cut out at rear for ball bearing arm supports
5 With provision for fitting tray.

Brakes

1 Paired brakes: both operated by a single left or right hand lever
2 Independent brakes
3 Brake lever extension for those who cannot reach standard brakes.

Cushions
Soft or hard
Depth between 1" (25.5 mm) and 4" (102 mm)
Soft upholstery on a plywood base is usually most comfortable
and can be removed for folding chair
A leathercloth covered foam cushion aids sliding transfers
Special paraplegic cushions are made to accommodate
urinals.

Special chairs
May be ordered if standard chairs are not suitable, e.g.
problems of space, transport or clinical conditions
One arm propulsion, semi-reclining, fully reclining position,
foot propulsion.

Electric indoor chairs
Patients who are not only unable to walk because of some
disability affecting the legs, but who, because of weakness
of their arms are also unable to propel themselves in an
ordinary wheelchair may be considered for an electrically
propelled indoor chair, only if this will help them to achieve
some measure of independence in the home, e.g.:
1 Tiller bar with lever control can be fitted to any Everest and
Jennings chair
2 Control box micro switch operation is mounted on either
side of the chair, can be positioned for the foot or mouth
control (child or adult)
3 "A.C. chair"; adult size only. Steering is leverset at either
side of chair and is power assisted.
Practical tests are needed to find the most suitable for each
patient
For further information consult D.H.S.S. Handbook of
Wheelchairs and Hand propelled tricycles or request
D.H.S.S. Technical officer in the area to visit patient at
home.

SUGGESTED FURTHER READING

Adams, J.C. (1978) *Outline of Fractures*. Edinburgh: Churchill Livingstone

Adams, J.C. (1977) *Outline of Orthopaedics*. Edinburgh: Churchill Livingstone

American Academy of Orthopaedic Surgeons (1966) *Joint Motion* Edinburgh: Livingstone

Daniels and Worthingham (1972) *Muscle Testing*. London: Saunders

Green, J. (1973) *Basic Clinical Physiology*. London: Oxford University Press

Houston, J.C., Joiner, C.L. & Trounce, J.R. (1975) *A Short Textbook of Medicine*. London: Hodder Educational

Jayson, M.I.V. & Dixon, A. St J. (1974) *Rheumatism and Arthritis*. London: Pan

Oxford Regional Health Authority (1978) *Equipment for the Disabled*. Oxford: ORHA

MacDonald, E.M. (1975) *Occupational Therapy in Rehabilitation*. London: Baillère Tindall

Moroney, J. (1975) *Surgery for Nurses*. Edinburgh: Churchill Livingstone

Sears, W.G. & Winwood, R.S. (1978) *Medicine for Nurses*. London: Arnold

Sinclair, D. (1975) *Introduction to Functional Anatomy*. Oxford: Blackwell

INDEX